LEARNING
TO CARE

LEARNING TO CARE

THE CARE HOME STAFF GUIDE

SUE BRAND

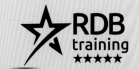

CONTENTS

FOREWORD

PROFESSOR MARTIN GREEN OBE
Chief Executive of Care England

Supporting people with complex needs is one of the most challenging, but also one of the most rewarding careers. Every day, staff working in care homes make a difference to people's lives, providing invaluable support and enabling them to live comfortably.

To do this job, you not only need the right values, but also the required skills and competencies. Once these are in place, you will be able to perform your role in the most supportive and safest way possible.

Built on the experience of the RDB Star Rating scheme, one of the most comprehensive and proven quality assurance systems, this book is full of useful and practical advice, which is presented in an incredibly clear and easy-to-follow way. The author, Sue Brand, draws on her extensive career for this essential guide, which meets the stringent requirements of regulation, allowing the reader to gain a deep understanding of what high-quality personalised care and support entails. Indeed, what differentiates this book from other resources is that it has been written by somebody whose experience of delivering care is second to none. The unique manner in which the book is written and the information it presents make it highly accessible to readers, as well as an invaluable training and development tool.

Working in the care sector can be demanding, but also incredibly satisfying. Once readers assimilate the information contained in this book, they will find themselves in the best place possible to deliver compliant and high-quality care. *Learning to Care: The Care Home Staff Guide* is an essential resource for care staff, and I commend it to everyone working in this sector.

M L Green

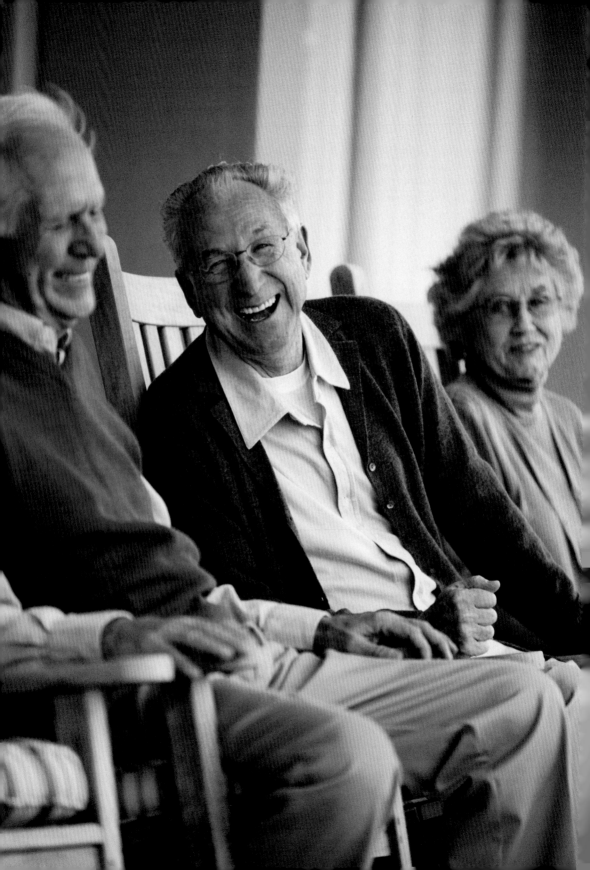

INTRODUCTION

Caring for people in their own home or a residential care home requires skill, commitment and knowledge. This can only be achieved by staff receiving pertinent, effective training to carry out this very important and challenging role.

So, what are the benefits of training?

- It will enable you to provide high-quality, compassionate care with dignity and respect.
- It will give you pride in your work, which will give increased job satisfaction.
- It will greatly benefit the person who you're caring for.

This training book is divided into three sections:

BEHAVIOURAL TRAINING

PRACTICAL TRAINING

FIRE TRAINING

1 BEHAVIOURAL TRAINING

The key qualities you need to be a good carer are empathy and compassion. Caring for vulnerable older people demands a great deal of sensitivity and understanding. For some people, age can bring wisdom, patience and tolerance, but for others it can bring depression, loneliness, pain, sorrow, humiliation, and a sense of loss and nostalgia for the past.

The Behavioural Training section of this book concentrates on how you should treat residents as individuals – understanding their problems, moods and sensitivities, while delivering high-quality care and services with dignity and respect.

The majority of older people know their limitations and are quite capable of knowing what is good and what is not good for them. They need to be treated with dignity as they deal with the frustration of growing old and developing progressive physical disabilities. It's intolerable if carers, family or friends treat them like children.

Carers must be resilient and approachable. They should not display an overprotective attitude towards residents, as this may adversely affect their health. If vulnerable older people cannot live their lives in the way they choose, they may feel there is no future and therefore no purpose in trying to cope with the many problems age brings. Eventually they may switch off and not participate in life at all.

If a carer, family member, friend or any other involved party becomes too authoritative, the pressure on a vulnerable person can cause them to make irrational decisions, which can have a devastating long-term effect on their lives. At no time must you assume that you know what is best for a person; this is an insult to their integrity and may be interpreted as patronising. Your job is to help and support vulnerable people to be as independent as they can, in the way that they choose.

2   PRACTICAL TRAINING

Age itself creates no restrictions; it is the malfunctioning of our bodies that creates them. This can happen at any age; some people are born with physical disabilities. However, it is only when we reach a certain age that physical disabilities appear to have another meaning. At this time, there is a danger of assuming that, as our bodies become frail and less active, our minds deteriorate at the same rate, and to the same level. This, of course, is not the case.

This section of the book covers practicalities such as dealing with residents' daily health and hygiene routines as well as the importance of getting the correct diagnosis for their symptoms. It also deals with emergencies, dehydration, falls, lifting techniques, mealtimes and nutrition, incontinence, dementia and confusion, and Covid-19.

3   FIRE TRAINING

Anyone who has experienced a fire, however small, will know just how frightening it can be, particularly if you are responsible for the care and wellbeing of others.

Two of the key reasons for deaths and injuries in a fire are when people panic or when staff do not know the correct procedures to follow.

INTRODUCTION

The act of controlling a fire is totally dependent upon the training that people receive in advance.

This section of the book, which is designed and written in particular for owners and staff in residential establishments of all kinds, including care homes, small hospitals, guest houses and hotels (although the same rules apply to educational institutions and commercial offices), provides staff with sound and practical advice on how to prevent and cope with a fire, should one break out in your care home, putting great emphasis on the correct procedures for staff to follow when the fire alarm sounds and before the fire brigade arrives.

WHAT NEXT?

During the Covid-19 pandemic in 2020/21, residents were much more vulnerable and needed their families to be at their side to give them comfort, reassurance and support but, due to lockdown restrictions, this was not always possible. The role of the carer, therefore, became even more important. What is the best way of coping in these unprecedented circumstances?

Once you have taken on board the advice in this book and can demonstrate the essential behavioural qualities and practical skills you need to be an outstanding carer, you can think about how you are going to polish your skills and develop yourself further. Caring for vulnerable people is a very rewarding and satisfying job. Make sure you take the time to learn and apply the lessons this book has to offer.

This training manual should be used as a reference book to frequently dip into, whenever you need clarification on a point you are not sure about. Read this book and discuss it with your manager and colleagues. We hope these guidelines will help you become even more professional in your job. Good luck!

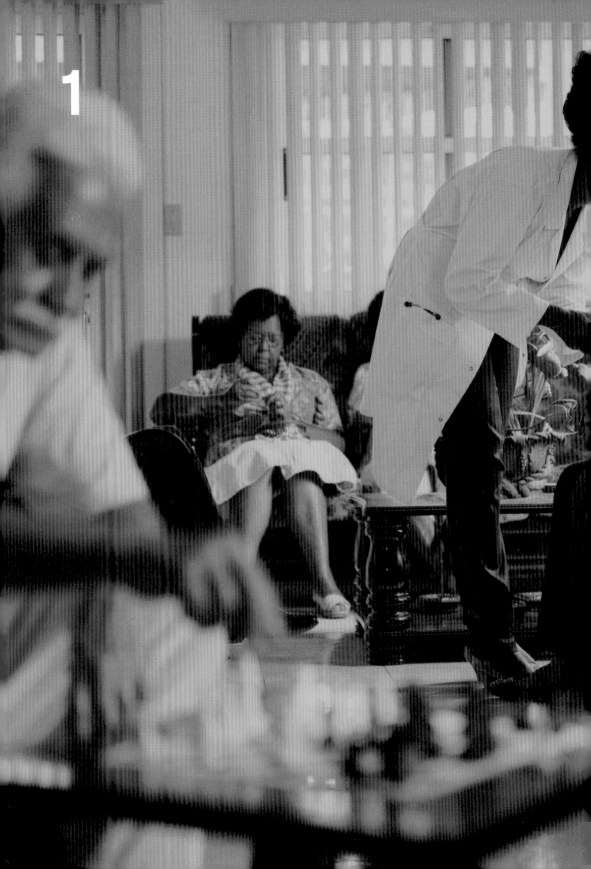

BEHAVIOURAL TRAINING

1 ABOUT THIS SECTION

This section is fairly short and easy to read. It's also one you should refer to time and time again, as things covered here often crop up in your job. Don't treat it as something you only read once and then forget about.

Why? Because it's there to help you, as a professional care assistant, to do your job better.

It's full of useful tips and advice. We haven't been able to include everything you'll ever need to know in your job, but you'll find that all the guidance it offers on how to care for your residents – and how they expect you to behave – will be very useful.

You're doing a very difficult but highly rewarding job. Make sure you take the time to learn and apply the lessons this book has to offer and polish your skills even further.

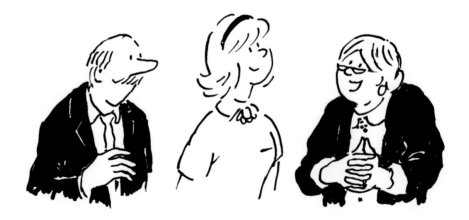

2   WHAT IS YOUR JOB?

That's easy to answer, isn't it? Your job is to 'care' for vulnerable people. But what does that mean?

It means you must be kind, compassionate and helpful, so, if you are considering becoming a care assistant you must already have these qualities. But there are additional qualities you need – patience, understanding, dedication and a heart of gold – oh, and a strong sense of humour too! Caring, and being cared for, is very much a two-way process between you and the resident.

Residents often say that they get their drive and enthusiasm from the staff. A happy, well-motivated team automatically creates a cheerful and positive environment; alternatively, a grumbling, fed-up and depressed staff team leaves residents feeling demoralised and depressed.

You will obviously bring your own personality into your work, which is essential. No two care assistants are alike in every detail and it is important that everybody can 'be themselves' in the job, without having to force themselves to behave differently.

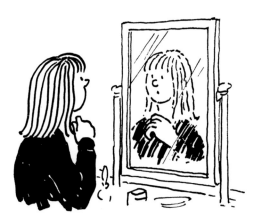

You need to ask yourself this: Why does a person go into a care home? What do they expect from the care home, and from you? Old age isn't an illness, it's a fact of life. It will happen to all of us sooner or later, if we are lucky. Unfortunately, too many people see old age as a condition where you get confused and forget things, fall over, can't walk, become incontinent, go blind and deaf, and complain all the time.

Now it's true that these things can happen to some people when they get older – but they don't automatically happen to everybody and they don't all happen to the same person. Some people live to a very ripe old age and never suffer from any of these problems. So really, the only difference between you and the average resident is that they are a bit older, and probably a bit wiser too.

So before committing yourself to this very rewarding and challenging job, it's important that you stop and think, to make sure in your own mind that you are the right kind of person to be a care assistant.

3 PUT YOUR BEST FOOT FORWARD

You'll find that you'll get on much better with the residents, and they'll get on much better with you, if you make the effort to put your best foot forward – especially in the way you look and dress.

Here are some of the areas to which you should pay particular attention:

CLOTHING

HANDS

GENERAL HYGIENE

3.1 CLOTHING

Clothing in some care homes can be quite casual, but it should be *clean* and well maintained. That includes shoes. There is nothing worse than seeing care assistants wandering around with grubby clothes on, buttons undone, or maybe missing, and clothes unironed.

If you take pride in your work, your appearance will reflect this. Seeing a scruffy care assistant tends to suggest that the person does not care much about what they are doing and gives the care home a bad image to residents and visitors.

3.2   HANDS

Hands are an important part of your job. You will be helping the residents with various functions, such as bathing, washing and doing up buttons, as well as handling and serving food. Your hands, therefore, are one of your essential tools of the trade.

Dirty fingernails are unpleasant, as well as unhygienic. Keep your nails trimmed and make sure that your hands are clean before tending to any of the residents, or handling food. Wear gloves and aprons if you are carrying out a resident's personal hygiene duties or particularly dirty jobs, and always wash your hands before and after each task.

3.3   GENERAL HYGIENE

Regular baths and showers are essential. No one wants to be looked after by a care assistant who has body odour. Some of the work you will undertake may be of a physical nature, such as hoisting people in and out of baths or bed, and this can cause a certain amount of perspiration. A daily bath or shower and a good deodorant should help to keep you fresh, but don't just use a deodorant instead of a bath or shower.

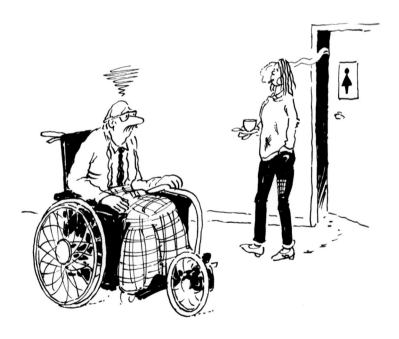

4 GOOD TIMEKEEPING

Residents like a regular daily routine. Things such as mealtimes are very important to them: they give each day a structure, and you must respect people's individual daily schedules. This is important for your work colleagues too.

If you are not good at timekeeping and are late on duty, someone has to cover for you until you arrive. Put yourself in their position – it is unreasonable of you to keep other members of staff from doing what they want to do or may have to do in their time off. You are part of a team, so make sure you are not the one who spoils the teamwork by being late on duty.

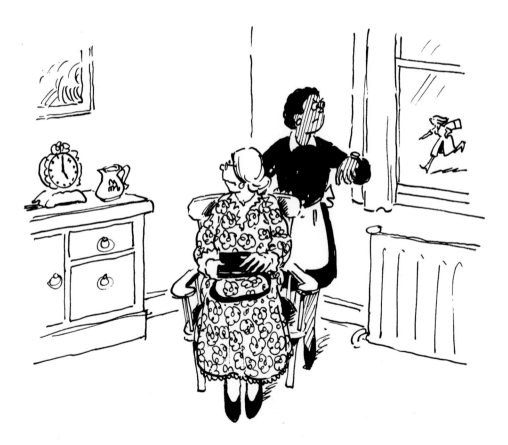

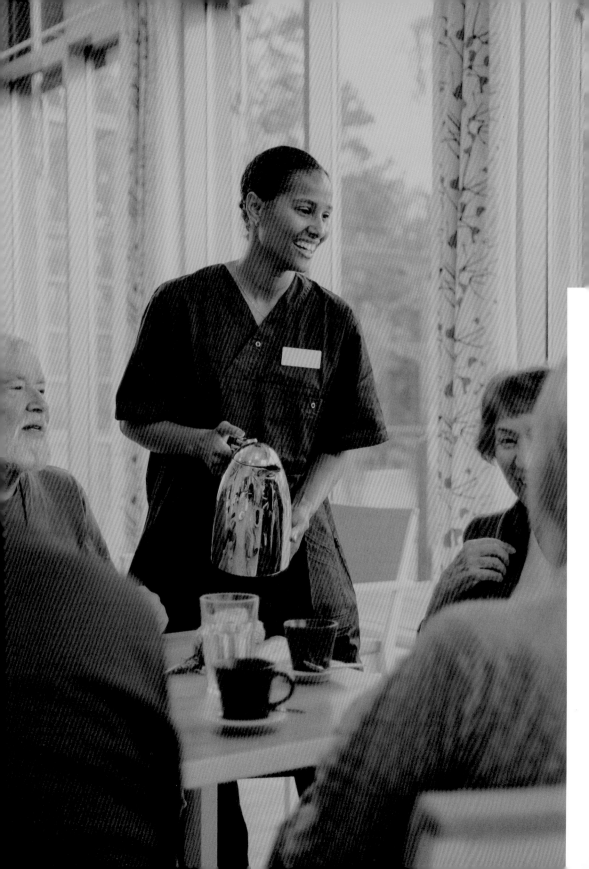

5   ANSWERING THE PHONE

Phones can sometimes be a nuisance, especially when you're busy on other duties. But they also have their uses: when the phone rings, it means that someone needs to communicate with the care home.

Answer the phone in a polite manner. Just picking it up and saying "Yes?" does nothing to enhance the reputation of the home. Use a friendly but business-like voice; it is always better to announce the name of the home rather than saying the number.

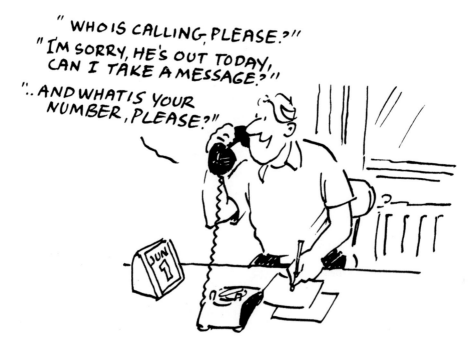

Listen carefully to what the caller has to say. If the call is for the manager, and they are not in the care home at the time, take a message. Make sure that you take the caller's correct name, number and message and repeat it to them to make sure it is correct. Note down the message immediately, otherwise, once you put the phone down and continue with your daily routine, you are likely to forget to pass the message on.

If the call is for a resident, ask for the name of the person speaking and relay the message correctly to the resident. If the resident is out or not available, ask if you can take a message. Again, make sure you write down the message immediately with the following information:

- the caller's name
- the caller's phone number
- the date and time of the call, and your initials.

Make sure that the correct person actually gets the message, whether that's by email, text or a note. Do not leave the message lying around on a table, where it may get lost or be picked up by someone else.

6 DEVELOPING THOSE SPECIAL QUALITIES

6.1 KEEP ON SMILING

Whatever the situation, the keyword is cheerfulness: don't be over-cheerful, unruly, loud or egotistical, but have a genuine cheerful and understanding air about you. Remember, a friendly, cheerful disposition rubs off; similarly, a grumpy, grudging personality not only shows, but may be mirrored by the resident. Make sure that your friendly disposition is genuine, not just a superficial smile. As the expression goes – smile from the heart – not the mouth.

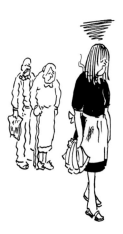 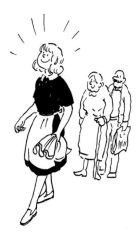

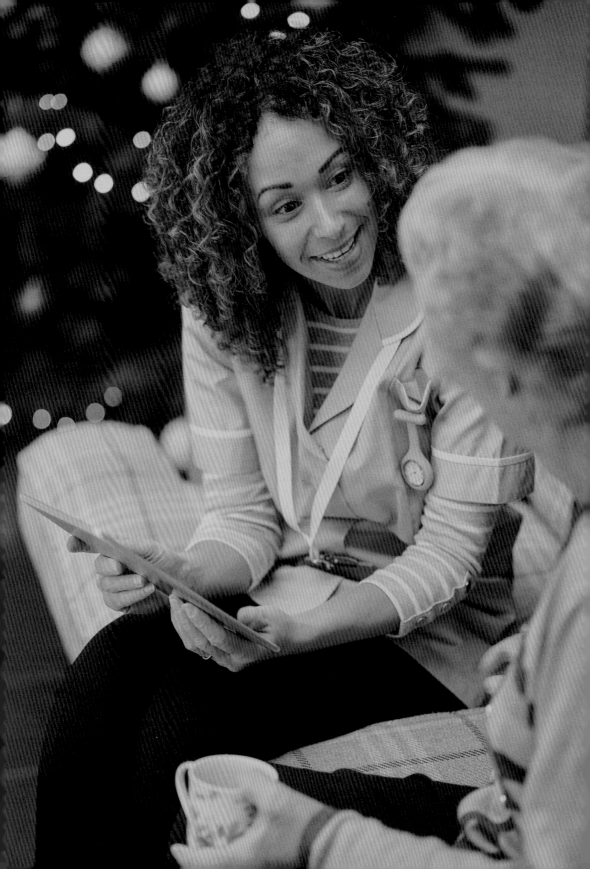

6.2 SHOW COMMITMENT

A care assistant needs to be totally committed to the role, so be flexible, as you will find there will be tasks that need to be done that are beyond your job description. You will have to help your colleagues and stand in for them when they are ill or off work, and be prepared to work at any time – weekends, holidays and even at Christmas. Being a care assistant is not just a job; it is a vocation.

6.3 SHOW THOUGHTFULNESS AND RESPECT

Care assistants should respect residents' wishes and allow them to be as independent as possible. Staff should encourage them to do things for themselves. Even if it does take longer, at least the resident will feel that they have achieved something.

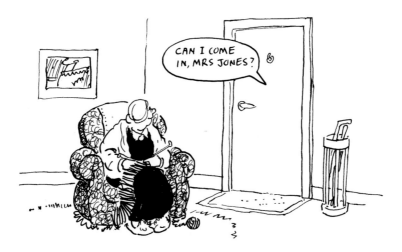

Remember, their room is part of their home now, so always knock on the door and wait for an answer before entering. Of course, if the resident is deaf, he or she may not have their hearing aid turned on, but knock anyway.

Respect their intelligence. Older people have a wealth of experience and some wonderful stories to tell. They tend to be more philosophical about life than the younger generation and therefore their comments and observations are very valued. Make the most of any spare moments you have to sit and talk to them; never use an excuse and say you are too busy.

23

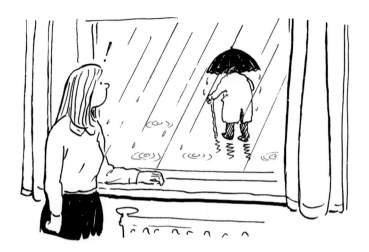

It is very difficult for residents who are physically disabled and have to come to terms with feeling young at heart but old in body. Many times, you will hear them saying how they would dearly love to go dancing, cycling or walking, if only their bodies would let them. It is very important to encourage, motivate and support these residents to keep active and mobile.

Respect their possessions; they may only have a few, but remember what they have brought into the care home with them are their most cherished. It can be very upsetting if you bang their ornaments down on a table, knock things over or damage something. However insignificant it may seem to you, it may become a major issue with them. The attitude you have towards their possessions will reflect on how you really feel about them.

Some of the following points will indicate to the resident whether you really respect their dignity:

- Do you address them how they wish? Would they like to be addressed by their first name or 'Mr/Mrs'? Use their preferred pronoun (she/he/they) too.
- Do you always knock on their door before entering?
- Do you help them with little tasks and give them a hand to get out of their chair or go to the toilet or commode without being asked?
- Do you remember their individual tastes and preferences?
- Does your understanding involve imagination? Residents like you to try not only to feel *for* them but *with* them.

- Do you have a sense of humour? A sense of humour can be of great value. If you help a person to laugh, you help them to live, and you get mutual satisfaction.
- Respect their privacy. With so many residents all strangers to one another living as a community, there may be some friction, particularly for people who are not very adaptable. Are you watchful and tactful?

6.4 DON'T ALWAYS WAIT TO BE ASKED

One of the problems with care assistant's role is that your duties never really finish. There is always something to be done or someone to help. Routine tasks can be planned and executed to a time schedule, but helping residents with all their little personal problems can never be planned.

Many residents do not like to ask a care assistant to help them to do simple jobs, for fear of being thought too demanding or a nuisance, so always reassure the person that's what you are there for. There are always jobs that residents will need some assistance with, such as writing letters, going for walks, sewing, or doing up buttons and zips. Remember, many may have poor eyesight, or their hands may be arthritic, so be observant and always lend a hand where you can.

Pay attention to detail and keep your eyes open for where your care may be needed, particularly with residents who are immobile or have problems with their sight. It's your job to check their toothbrush, flannel, and brush and comb do they need to be cleaned or replaced? Does an item of clothing need to be washed or mended?

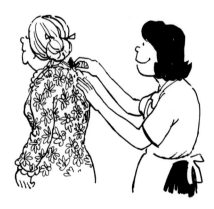

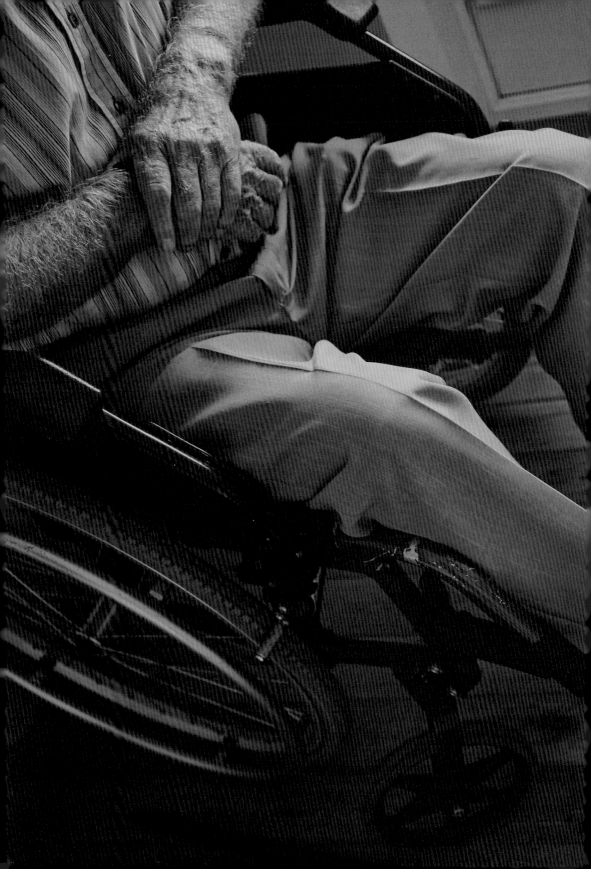

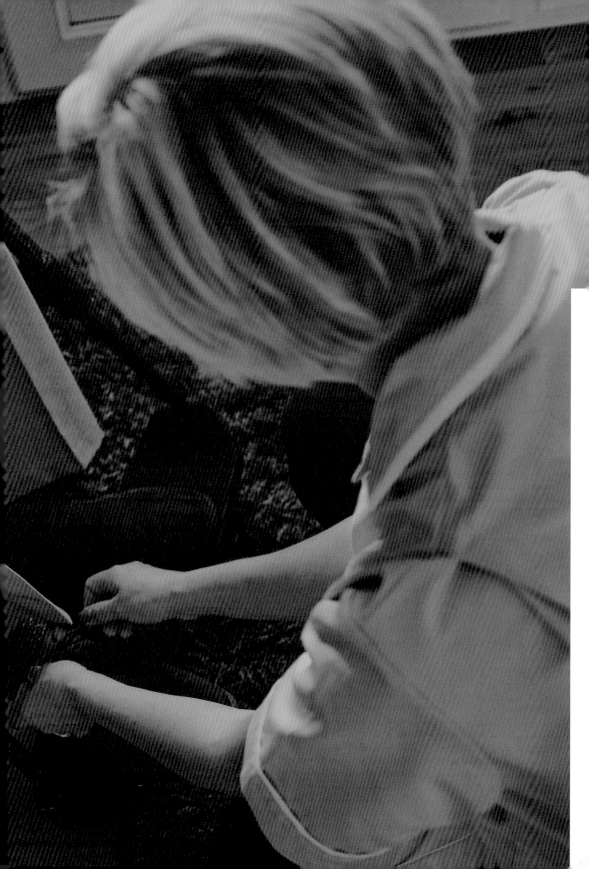

6.5   SHOW DISCRETION

We are all discreet, or we like to think we are, but in a care home the need for discretion is of paramount importance. It can make the difference between a contented, relaxed atmosphere and a home where people distrust each other and are edgy. Keep your eyes and ears open to what is going on around you and approach all situations with discretion.

Another important point to remember is that you should never discuss your personal problems with residents; they have enough to worry about already. If you have personal or family problems of your own, discuss them with your manager.

One of the most important aspects of keeping harmony in a care home is to be loyal to the people you come into contact with in the home. Never discuss or criticise any member of staff or resident with any other member of staff or resident, and remember that you must always report any complaints, concerns or observations to your manager.

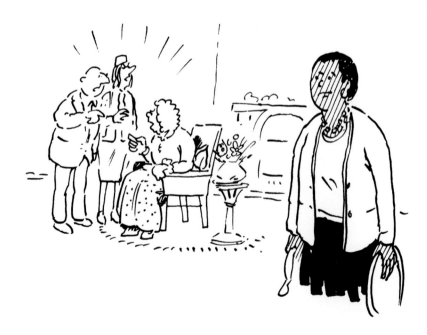

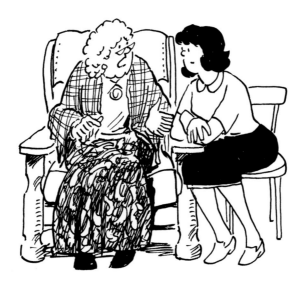

6.6 SHOW UNDERSTANDING

Many elderly people dwell on the past and reflect on the 'good old days'. This is understandable because their past is their *life*, and they gain comfort from their fond memories and past experiences. It is a fact that many people can remember more vividly things that happened, say, 20 or 30 years ago than a few weeks or days ago, and they usually remember the good times, not the bad. Residents enjoy telling staff about their lives, so it is important for you to be a good listener.

Understanding the issues facing elderly people has several aspects. For some, age may bring wisdom and dignity, but for others it may bring loneliness and ill health. Some suffer humiliation, particularly if they are very dependent on staff for help with all their personal needs. The care assistant must react with understanding and sensitivity in these situations.

Problems that may seem trivial to you may loom large in their minds. A dripping tap or breakfast being late can upset their whole day. Make sure you handle all their problems and troubles quickly, efficiently and with understanding.

If a resident appears down or in a bad mood, spend time talking to them and try to find out what the matter is. Remember, you are probably in the best position to help. Sometimes we all feel in a low mood for no apparent reason, so expect this from the residents as well. This is their home, so they can't get away and have their mood in private – you can.

Maintain trust if a resident discusses a confidential matter with you and do not divulge it to others. If, on the other hand, you think your manager should know, as the person appears very distressed and upset, ask their permission to discuss it with the manager.

Do not treat all residents the same. They are all different and like to be treated as such, so know their sensitivities and act accordingly, and never show favouritism. This is what makes the care assistant's job so interesting and stimulating and ensures that the care home is relaxed and friendly.

- Always treat residents with compassion, dignity and respect.
- Be positive and maintain a cheerful, friendly manner.
- Make them feel welcome: it is their home.
- Make sure that all residents keep fit and well and support them to keep their independence and mobility as far as possible, bearing in mind any difficulties they may have, such as arthritis.
- Respect the residents' privacy, and never patronise them or treat them like children.
- Avoid having favourites, however difficult this may be.
- Avoid showing irritation or annoyance with a strong-minded or difficult resident.

7 UNDERSTANDING RESIDENTS' BEHAVIOUR

None of us are perfect, so you may find that occasionally you have 'personality problems' with a resident. This could be for any number of reasons. You may find a resident is particularly 'awkward' – but they may *always* have been awkward. Others may have problems adjusting to life in the care home.

Here are just a few types of personality traits to consider:

- the resident you will never please
- the troublemaker
- the carping critic
- the complainer
- the aggressive type

- the gossip
- the dictator
- the hypochondriac
- the disrupter
- the selfish type

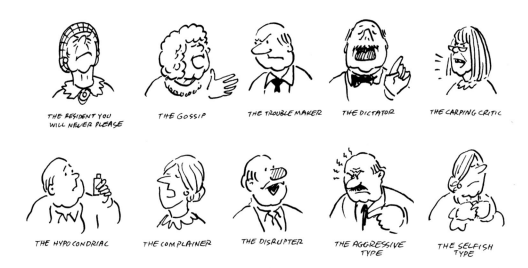

THE RESIDENT YOU WILL NEVER PLEASE

THE GOSSIP

THE TROUBLE MAKER

THE DICTATOR

THE CARPING CRITIC

THE HYPOCONDRIAC

THE COMPLAINER

THE DISRUPTER

THE AGGRESSIVE TYPE

THE SELFISH TYPE

Dealing with people who exhibit these traits is not easy. Experience, understanding and a professional, friendly approach will help. Never lose your patience or get irritated. Remember, it takes two to make an argument. Once the resident knows that it is no use, for example, gossiping to you, or being aggressive with you, then they are more likely to desist. They may try it on your colleagues, but then it is up to them to overcome the problem.

The biggest challenge of your job is to understand why, when you believe you are kind, thoughtful and caring, a resident does not respond, but continually complains and criticises. Unfortunately, it is not always possible to diagnose these traits beforehand, and it is a part of your job that you will have to learn to deal with. You must accept the fact that you are not going to please all the people all of the time. The professional care assistant will be able to identify those residents who have a genuine complaint, and those who just enjoy complaining.

It takes time and experience to deal with these situations. Do remember that residents are paying for your assistance, and some believe they therefore have the privilege of finding fault and complaining.

Should you be unable to cope with a situation or if you believe that one resident is annoying others, then you must immediately inform your manager.

8   DEALING WITH CONFUSION

We all get confused and forgetful at times, particularly when we are stressed, but when we are young, we do not use 'age' as an excuse. It is a mistake to assume that age is responsible for everything: this gives very little hope to the older person. Remember that old age is *not an illness*. Residents are likely to appear 'confused' to some extent sooner or later, but nothing is inevitable, and staff can play a vital role in keeping a resident from becoming permanently confused.

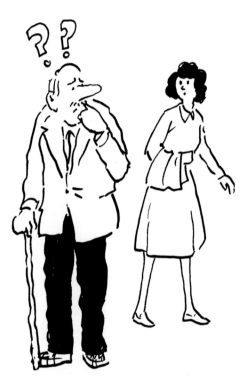

If a resident suddenly appears 'confused' for no apparent reason, seek medical advice immediately. Do not let it go unchecked. When this happens, reassure the resident, try to find out if they have any problems, or whether they are unhappy in the home. Perhaps their friends or family do not come and visit as often as they would like. Spend time with them: they will feel very frightened, because dementia is what most people dread more than anything. Reassure them that suddenly becoming confused does not mean it will be permanent.

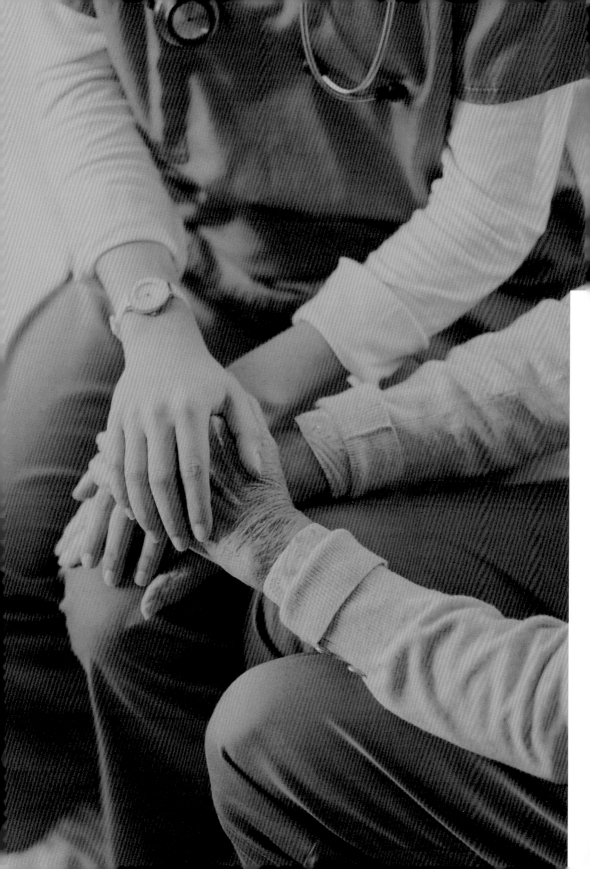

There are various causes of confusion, and these need to be ruled out:
- Has the resident been prescribed any new drugs lately?
- Are they dehydrated?
- Do they have a urine infection?
- Are they eating properly?
- Are they drinking (alcohol) and taking sleeping tablets and tranquillisers at the same time?
- Do they have an underlying illness?
- Do they have a deep psychological problem that they will not discuss?

During their period of temporary confusion:
- Never lead them on to believe that they have dementia.
- Never reprimand or scold them.
- Never laugh at them or make fun of them.
- Never ignore the symptoms.
- Always report it to your manager.
- Always seek medical help.

If tests are carried out and the correct treatment is given, the resident will probably soon return to normal health and stop being confused. Your special care during this period is essential.

9   THE ROLE OF OCCUPATIONAL THERAPY

Occupational therapy relieves boredom and stimulates mental and physical abilities. It is essential that elderly people have some sort of occupation to stimulate and motivate them – and of course they should be encouraged to continue the hobbies they've always had.

If they don't have interests already, encourage residents to take up some kind of work, maybe knitting or sewing or helping with something in the home, for example laying tables or folding napkins. Whatever work the resident undertakes, there must be a genuine need for the finished article: for example, baby clothes for the hospital or blankets for charities. Residents will become annoyed and demotivated if they believe that they have just been asked to undertake a task to keep them occupied.

Residents should also be encouraged to become involved in the community so that they do not become isolated and cut off from everyday life. Contact with neighbours and strangers from the locality

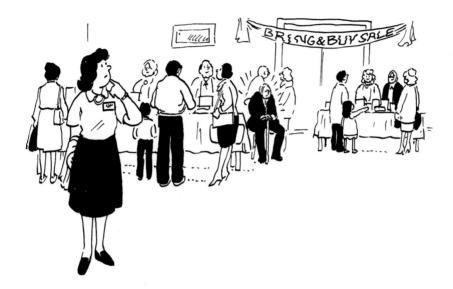

leads to a feeling of belonging. Arrange outings if possible, or afternoon teas, and a bring-and-buy stall. This creates many different jobs to be undertaken, such as serving teas, working on the door, and manning various stalls. It also gives residents a chance to chat with people who come along to buy. Planning and advertising an event can also create opportunities for residents to get involved, and they will have something to talk about between themselves, with staff and of course, with their relatives and friends when they visit.

10   THE NEW RESIDENT

New residents in particular need your understanding. Over the past few months their world has most likely been turned upside down. They may have lost a spouse or been ill. The decision to go into a care home may have been forced on them by their family or because of medical pressures. They most likely will be giving up the home where they have lived for many years, with all its memories. The anguish and distress caused by having to sell their home and give away their furniture and treasured possessions will inevitably leave them drained and in a state of shock by the time they arrive at the care home.

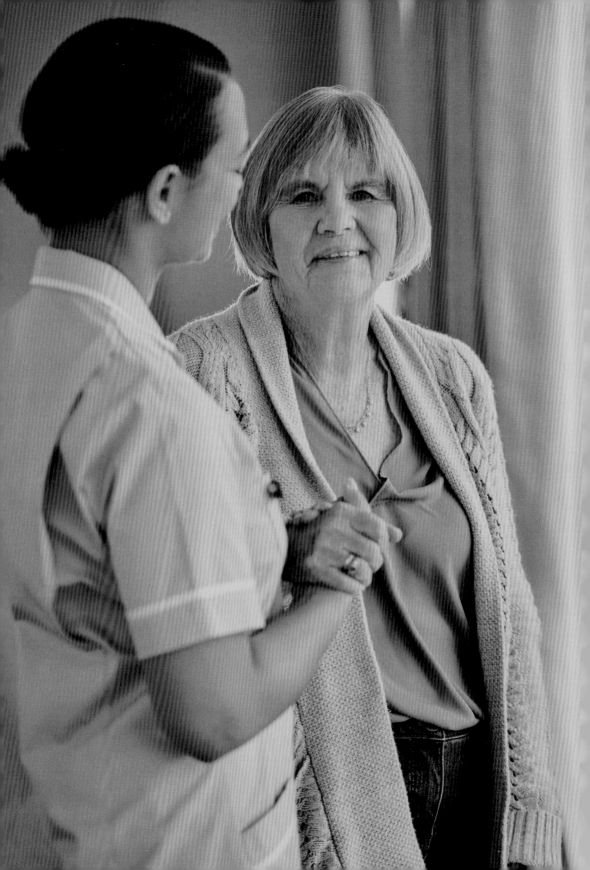

Because of the traumatic events they may have suffered prior to arrival, it is not unusual for new residents to appear confused and disorientated, or even to be incontinent. Usually a good night's sleep, good food, and kind and caring staff is all they need to put them on the right road again. It takes about three months for a resident to begin to feel 'at home'; during this period, they will be wondering whether or not they have made the right decision. It is therefore important for a prospective resident to come to the care home for a month's trial period, before making the very difficult decision to move in permanently.

If a resident does not like their environment, then they may become aggressive or 'switch off'. The care assistant should make sure that this does not happen. All staff must be very understanding, sympathetic and reassuring. Kindness at a time like this can play a crucial part in the future wellbeing and contentment of the resident. Patience and understanding during this final decision period is not too much for the resident to ask for, and not too much for care assistants to give.

A resident's confusion and incontinence could well become permanent if they feel the staff:

- are impatient about their inability to adjust quickly
- appear not to understand why they feel miserable
- do not listen to their concerns or problems
- ignore their 'cries for help'.

11   HANDLING VISITORS TO THE HOME

There are two main categories of visitors to the care home:

OFFICIAL VISITORS

RESIDENTS' FAMILIES AND GUESTS

11.1   OFFICIAL VISITORS

You will come into contact with various authorities. They regularly visit care homes to make sure that residents are safe in your care and that regulations are being adhered to. They are *not* there to catch you out.

They want to ensure that you are delivering safe, high-quality care and services with compassion, dignity and respect.

You can expect to be asked questions, which you should answer in a polite and direct manner. If you are not sure of the answer, say so, and direct them to the manager. Never try to 'fudge' an answer – they will pick that up very quickly. The main people visiting are likely to be:

- from the Care Quality Commission (CQC) – the body that regulates care homes
- GPs and pharmacists
- from the social services department of the local authority
- from the Health and Safety Executive
- from the fire brigade.

11.2   RESIDENTS' FAMILIES AND GUESTS

Residents like to see relatives and guests – it gives them something to look forward to.

When visitors arrive, make them feel welcome and at ease. Contact the resident, tell them who has arrived and ask them where they would like to see them: in the lounge, garden or in their room.

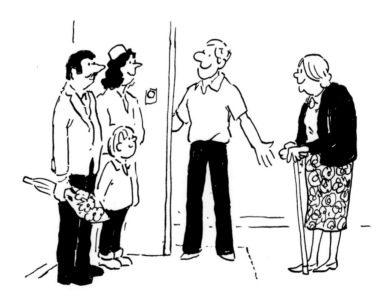

If you know guests are going to be visiting, help the resident with any last-minute preparations such as dressing, cleaning or tidying up. Should guests bring flowers or fruit, offer to give them a vase or fruit bowl if the resident doesn't have one handy.

Guests should feel happy about the resident being in your care home. They should leave feeling that the resident is being well cared for and is contented. Don't put on a facade to try to impress guests, because the residents will think you are being false. Be yourself – concerned, caring and good natured.

12 EQUALITY, DIVERSITY AND INCLUSION

The home's Statement of Purpose will include the aims and philosophies that promote equality and diversity in your workplace. Your manager has a duty to ensure that services are delivered in a way that is fair, personalised and diverse to meet the needs of all the residents. You, as a care assistant, have a responsibility to treat everyone equally, whether they are residents or other colleagues, and not to stereotype and/or discriminate against individuals or groups on the basis of their age.

Within your role as a care assistant, you should always do your best to:

- promote these values throughout your role
- ensure you treat residents fairly and equally, with dignity and respect
- understand and respect the needs and wishes of each resident
- not be judgemental of residents or colleagues' beliefs or religions.

It is important to remember that residents rely on you to provide a lot of their care and to look after them in a way that they no longer can. Since this is a key part of your role, you must understand how people's background, culture and community can influence their past experiences, future aspirations, relationships, and their care and support needs.

In your role, you may come across values or beliefs that are very different to yours, on religion, sexual orientation or politicals. It is your job to put those differences aside and deliver high-quality and compassionate care with respect for the individual.

12.1 INCLUSION

Living in a care home is very much like living at home in the community. The care home and the residents' room becomes their home and the other residents become like neighbours, just like when they were living at home, so most residents want to feel included in what is going on around them. It is important for you to make sure that you are working in an inclusive way, ensuring that all residents feel they are included in the running of the home.

This means that you must:

- offer them all the same choices
- ensure you give all residents the same opportunities
- not exclude residents from activities
- always assume that a resident wants to be included in something.

13 YOU AND THE MANAGEMENT

Your relationship with your manager is very important, as are your relationships with other members of staff.

Your manager's duty is to ensure that the residents always come first and that the care home runs smoothly and efficiently.

Should you have any problems with your duties and assignments, talk to your manager. Do not bottle things up and complain to other members of staff. It is much better to arrange an appointment with your manager to discuss it with him or her.

Staff are responsible for the smooth running of the home. If people do not carry out their jobs properly, then problems happen, disruption is caused, and the residents suffer. Your manager has worked out duties and timetables to cover all foreseeable eventualities; some, however, can be unforeseen, such as staff illness or accidents. You may therefore be called upon to undertake extra duties and functions at short notice. Remember that if you are sick, someone must cover for you, so be prepared to do the same for them.

Do not treat your relationship with your manager as 'us and them'. You are employed at the home as a care assistant, and you and your manager are there to make the residents' lives enjoyable and fulfilling. A friendly, informal relationship between staff will help everyone retain a warm atmosphere in the home.

Respect for your manager must always be maintained. Some managers like you to use their first names, some do not, but whatever the situation, a friendly, open and relaxed atmosphere is essential.

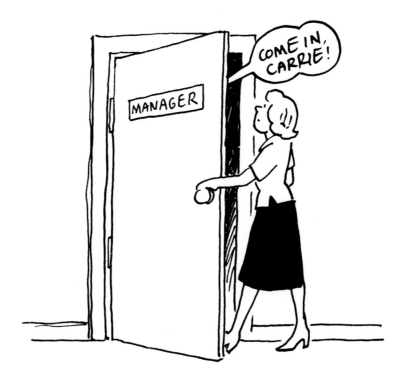

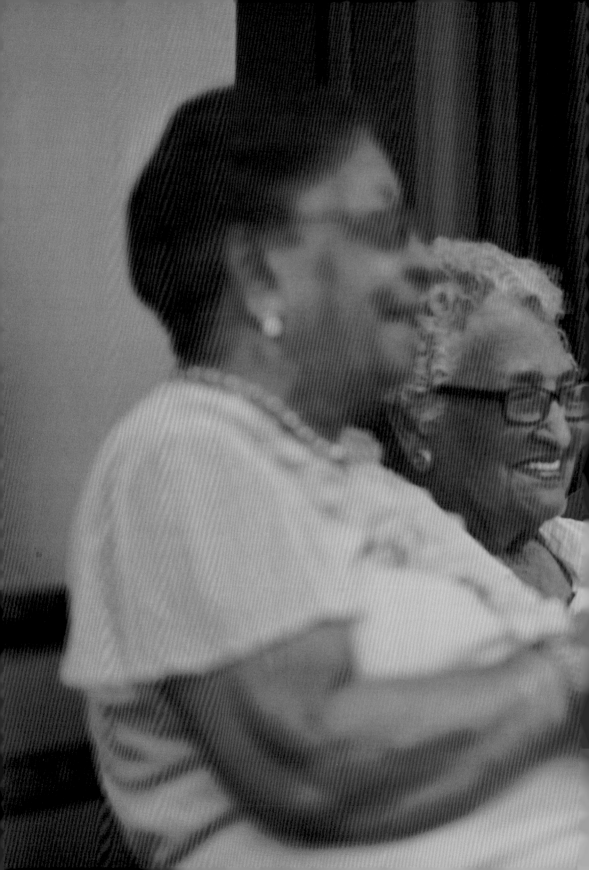

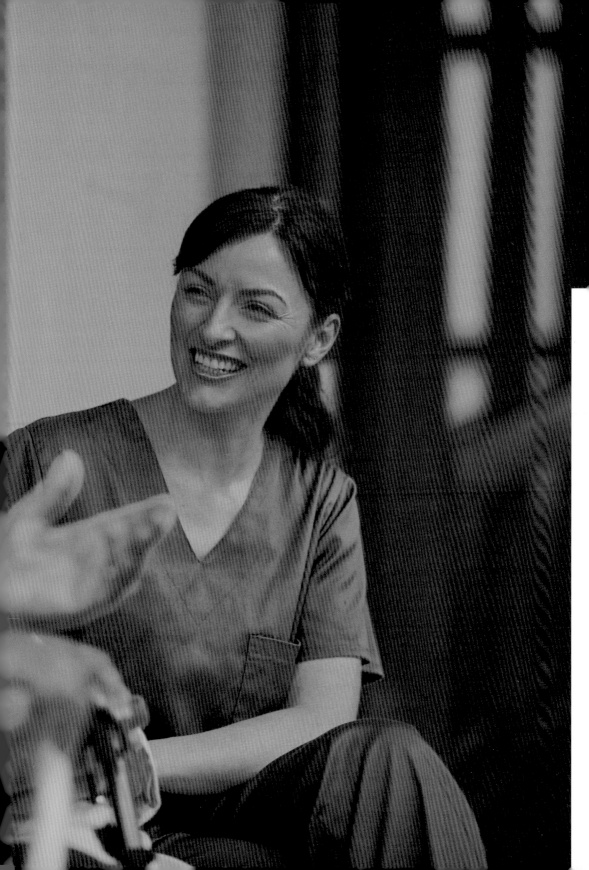

NOTES

M	T	W

T	F	S / S

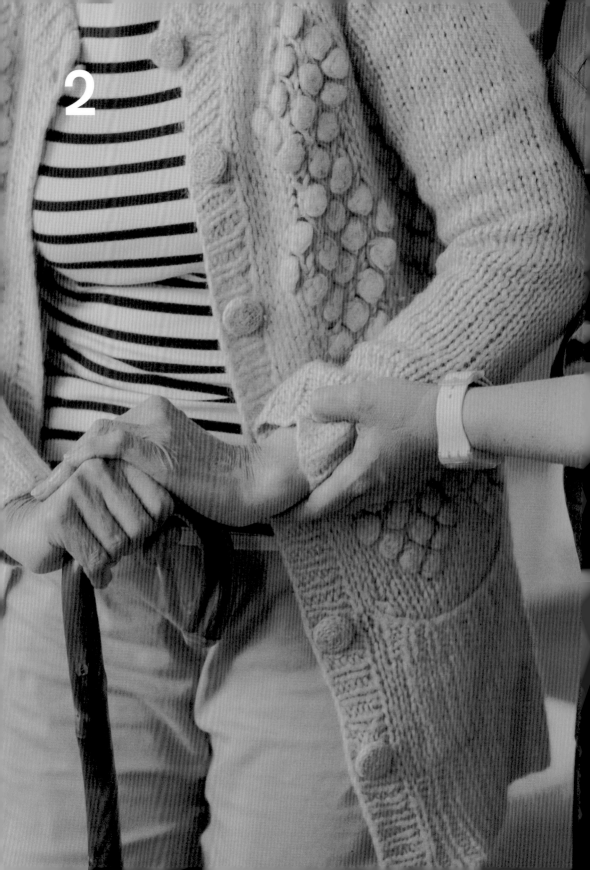

PRACTICAL TRAINING

1   WHAT IS YOUR JOB?

There are many different demands placed on you as a care assistant in a care home. Nobody expects you to have the detailed knowledge and skills a nurse would have, but you should be able to give the level of care that a loving relative would.

The ages of residents in a care home can range from 18 upwards and you must treat everyone as individuals. Your job is to help residents to be as independent as possible and encourage them to do as much as they can for themselves, but you'll need to give extra care to residents who are more frail or disabled than others. Residents like a basic routine so they can organise their daily lives. They like their meals, baths and their room cleaned on time so they can plan their day.

In this section of the book, you will find some useful practical guidance on how to improve your residents' quality of life.

2   RESIDENTS' DAILY CARE PLANS

In helping your residents to take good care of themselves, you must make sure you provide the care recorded in their individual care plans, which may be electronic or on paper.

A senior member of staff develops the care plan with the involvement of the resident and/or their representative when they first arrive at the care home. The care plan details the resident's wishes on how their care and services should be delivered. It is a working document which is regularly reviewed and updated and covers all aspects of a resident's health, care and wellbeing. Care plans include the following:

• Their preferences for how they wish to live their lives
• Their current care and treatment
• Dietary assessments and requirements
• Difficulties with eating, drinking or swallowing
• Mobility assessments and equipment
• Social activities
• End-of-life care.

Care plans contain details of each resident's health and behaviour: therefore, you need to read them before you start your shift and write them up when you finish your shift. This way the staff who come on duty for the next shift will know exactly what's been going on and what to do, such as whether Mrs A has become a great-grandmother yet, or how Mrs B is coping with the flu. All these things, however trivial they may seem to you, should be recorded. Your manager also reads your notes to keep in touch with the goings-on in the home.

Anything that you consider important or different from the daily happenings should also be reported verbally to your manager or a senior member of staff.

There are lots of things that you need to do to look after your residents properly, and you must know how to do them well.

But remember, every shift starts and ends with the care plans.

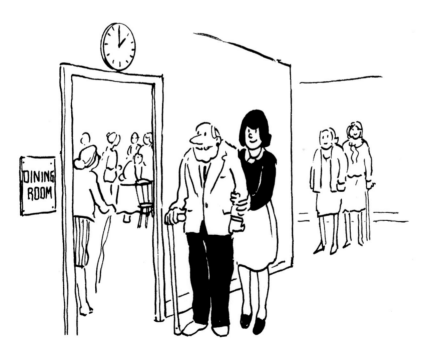

3 TAKING GENERAL CARE OF RESIDENTS' HEALTH

On your daily rounds of bed making, bathing and serving drinks and meals, you must keep an eye on the health of the residents. Make time to sit and talk, particularly to the lonely, who have very few visitors, and the depressed. Try to encourage them and cheer them up. A cheerful smile works wonders.

Some of the signs of ill health are bad sleeping patterns, loss of appetite, a feeling of lethargy and any change in behaviour. These should be reported to your manager and recorded in the resident's care plan. The resident must then be monitored for a day or two to see if their condition improves or deteriorates. If a resident does not feel well, but does not feel ill enough to call the doctor:

- Take their pulse and temperature and write these down.
- Talk to them to find out exactly how they feel, if they are in any pain or have any specific symptoms.
- Find out if they are anxious or worried about anything.
- Find out if they have been prescribed any new medication recently.

Make sure that all the answers are reported to your manager and recorded in the resident's care plan.

Always be available to listen to a resident's or their family's complaints or problems, and make sure you do something about them. If the solution is beyond you, report it to your manager and follow it through to make sure that the resident and their family are satisfied.

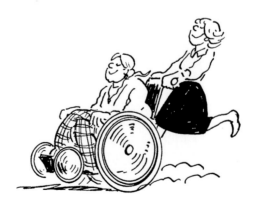

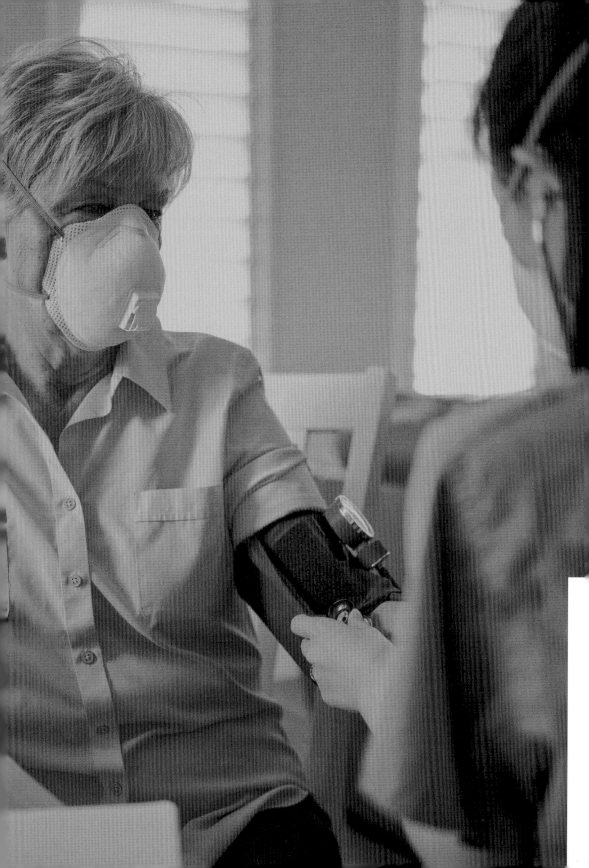

4 THE DAILY HOUSEHOLD ROUTINE

A care home is a home and like any other home, there are lots of little domestic jobs that have to be done every day. Because the residents are a little older than most of us, some aspects of the daily routine have to be handled with more care.

4.1 BED MAKING

Don't tuck sheets and blankets too tightly, or the bed will be difficult to get into.

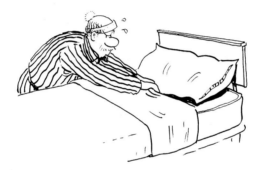

4.2 HELP WITH DRESSING AND UNDRESSING

Take care when helping residents to dress or undress, so you don't injure someone or hurt their pride.

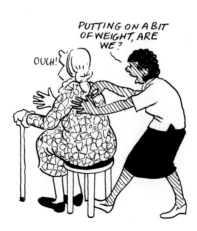

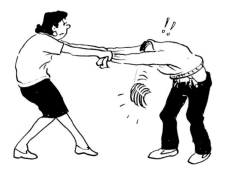

4.3   HELPING WITH BATHING

Always make sure the temperature of the water is right for each resident by using a temperature probe.

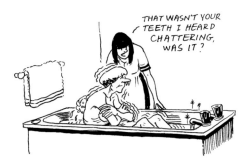

4.4   HELPING WITH WASHING

Consider the resident's privacy and dignity at all times.

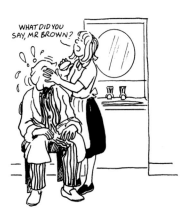

4.5   LAUNDRY

Always take care of residents' clothes.

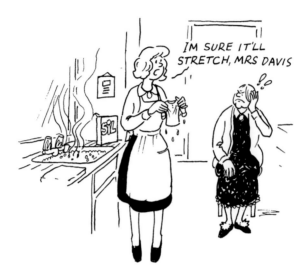

4.6   PREPARATION OF RESIDENTS' TRAYS FOR MEALS AND DRINKS

Know all your residents' likes, dislikes, allergies and nutritional requirements.

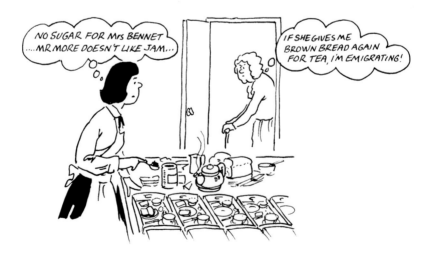

60

4.7 **TEMPERATURE AND PULSE TAKING**

Always concentrate on the job in hand.

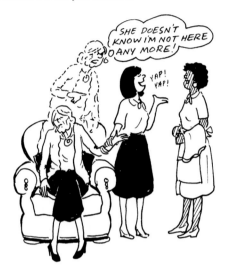

4.8 **HELPING WITH PERSONAL THINGS**

For more dependent or immobile residents, you will also be responsible for keeping all their personal things in order. Their brushes and combs should be cleaned regularly, and face flannels washed daily. Chests of drawers and wardrobes should be kept clean and tidy, so that residents can easily find the clothes they are looking for, and many residents will need your help in maintaining their personal appearance.

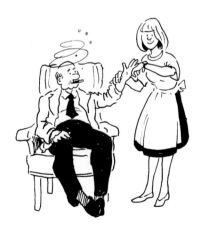

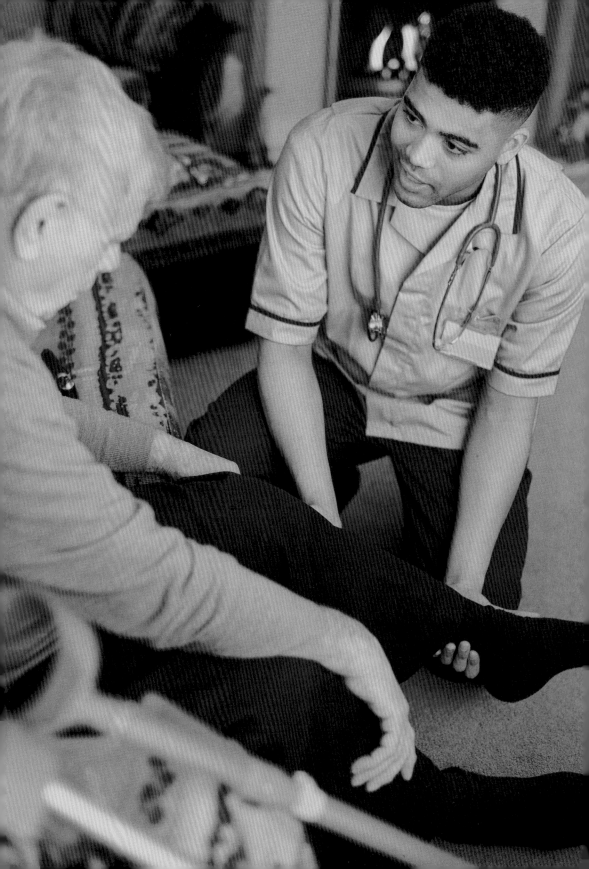

5 MOVING AND HANDLING RESIDENTS

You must received training before you attempt to lift someone. The two important rules here are quite simple:

PROTECT THE RESIDENT

PROTECT YOURSELF.

5.1 PROTECT THE RESIDENT

A resident who needs lifting is going to feel vulnerable, so they must feel confident when you lift them or they will become distressed and the lifting process will be made even more difficult. They may also, of course, get hurt.

5.2 PROTECT YOURSELF

If you don't know what you are doing, you not only run the risk of injuring the resident, but you may well get hurt too. There are two rules to think about when lifting, which will help you protect the resident and yourself.

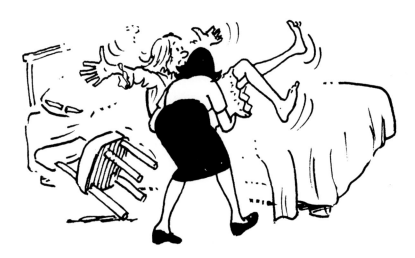

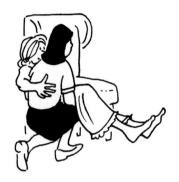 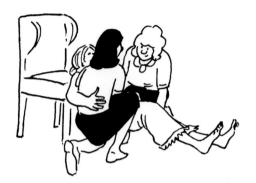

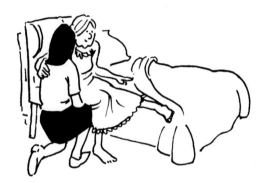 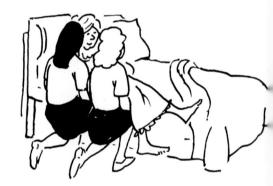

Always remember, whether you are assisting someone or you're on your own: *bend your knees and keep your back straight.*

A damaged back will cause you pain. As a result:

- Your state of mind, your concentration and your temper will suffer.
- You physically won't be able to do your job properly and you may have to take time off work.
- Your employer will have to get someone else to cover for you.
- The residents will have to get to know someone new.
- You will be miserable.

So remember *lifting* can be *dangerous.* Learn how to do it *before* you *have* to, and always get someone else to help you.

6 TEETH, EARS AND EYES

6.1 TEETH

Many of the residents will wear dentures, so there are several things that you must watch for:

- that the dentures fit properly
- that the dentures are kept clean
- that the resident is always given their own, not someone else's! (This may sound funny, but you'd be surprised how often it happens.)

If you do not take special care here, the resident may get:

- sore gums and possibly even ulcers
- frustrated because they cannot eat properly
- frustrated because they cannot speak properly
- depressed
- angry.

If you notice any of these problems, record it in the resident's care plan and report it to your manager, who will make an appointment for the resident to see the dentist. Do not let it go unchecked.

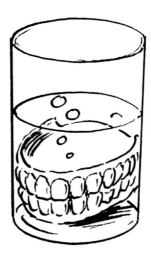

6.2 EARS

Hearing plays a very important part in a resident's communication with family, other residents and staff. If a resident cannot hear properly, they may reply to questions with completely the wrong answers, which may make people think they are confused or have dementia. This in turn may lead the resident to become depressed and withdrawn. Some people are not aware of how impaired their hearing is, so if you have any doubts about a resident's hearing, report it to the manager, who will discuss it with the resident's GP.

Often the problem is caused by something as simple as having wax in the ears, which can soon be put right. If the resident owns a hearing aid, make sure that they can work it properly and have a supply of batteries.

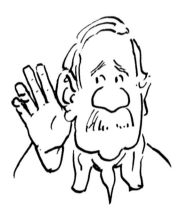

6.3 EYES

Anyone complaining of failing vision needs to have an eye test. Many elderly people find the quality of their vision changes as the years pass, even though their eyes appear normal.

A change could also be due to cataracts, glaucoma or other eye pathology. A visit to the local opticians is advisable. As well as carrying out an eye test, they will also check for any abnormalities of the eyes. If they find any problems, they will notify the resident's GP.

It is important to remember that none of us can see in the dark. Older people must have good lighting and should have an anglepoise lamp for reading and all close work. The light should come from over their shoulder. A ceiling light or standard lamp is adequate. Reading of small print can be helped with the use of handheld magnifying lenses, which are available from most opticians.

People complaining of difficulty with vision should always have their sitting room arranged so that their armchair has its back to the window, allowing the light to come from behind the resident. For the same reason, the television should be positioned away from the window. When walking outside, residents may find it helpful to wear a hat with a brim to shade the sun, or a sun visor.

Blind and partially sighted people need special help. It is most important to remember that nothing in their room should be moved without their permission. Not only will moving things upset them, but it can cause confusion and possibly accidents as well. Everything should have an established place in their room.

People who are registered as blind or partially sighted may be eligible for special help from social services.

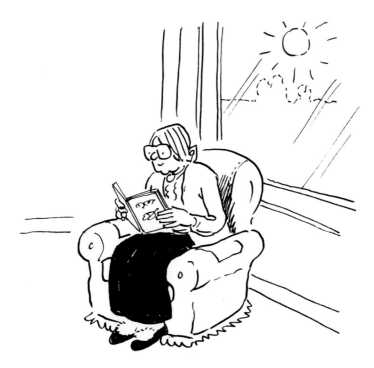

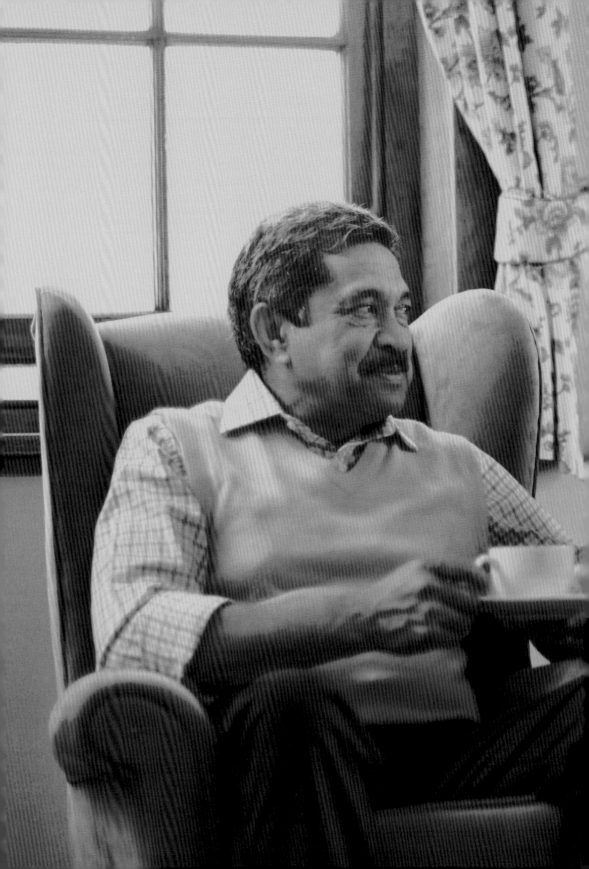

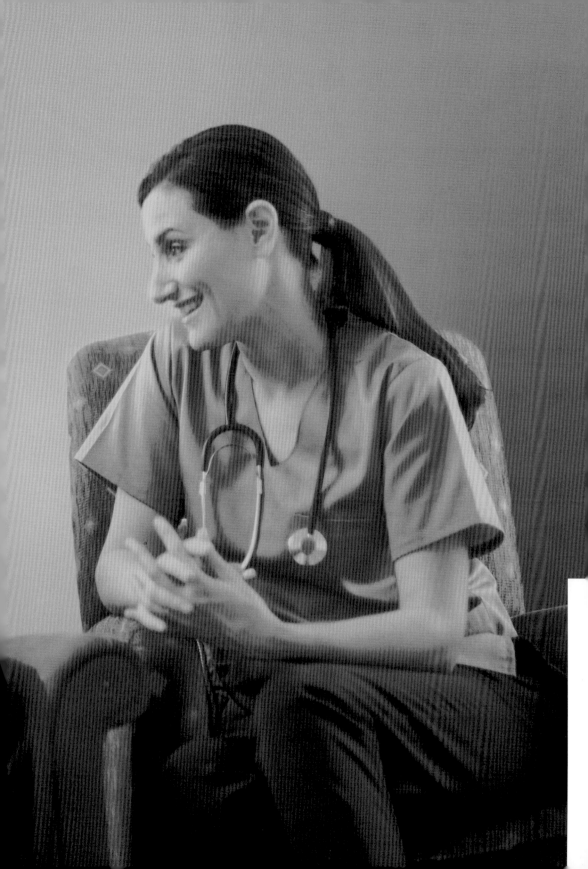

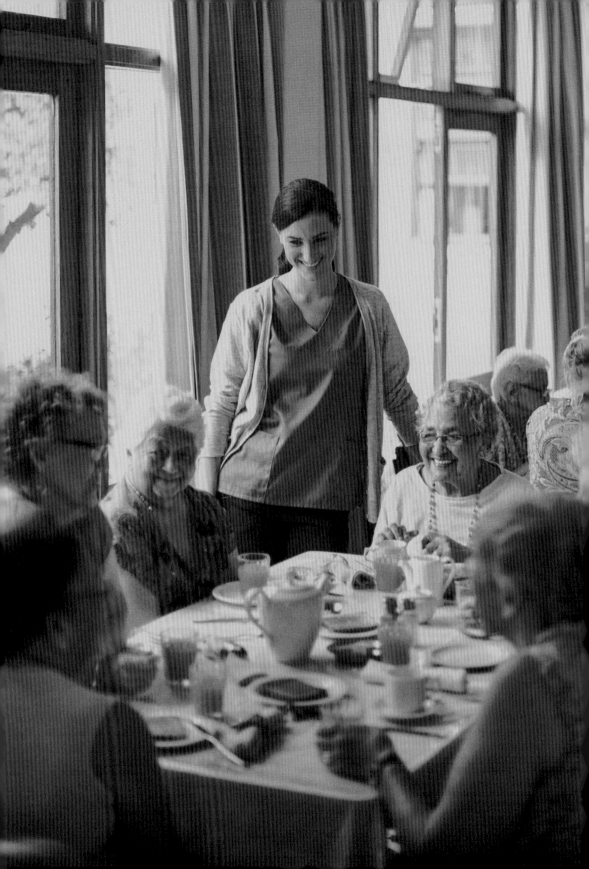

7   MEALS, MEALTIMES AND NUTRITION

Care assistants have a duty to the residents to make sure that mealtimes are as pleasant and enjoyable as possible. They also have a duty to observe if any resident has a problem with eating, which you must record in the resident's care plan and report to your manager.

Nutrition plays a key role in the lives of residents, not only in keeping them fit and healthy, but also it is the one area that the residents can judge for themselves how much the home and the staff really care about their health and wellbeing.

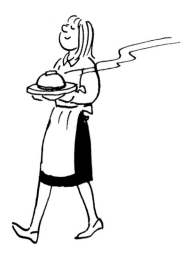

Here is a checklist of some of the points that residents will notice:

- Is the food well presented and tasty?
- Is the food served hot or lukewarm?
- Are residents given the correct portion for their individual appetites?
- Has any thought gone into menu planning to provide varied and interesting meals, or are they monotonous and dull?
- Are the residents' favourite dishes included in the menus?
- Is there a choice of menu if a resident doesn't like what is being served?
- Are mealtimes flexible, or are the times organised for the benefit of the staff, not the residents?
- Do the staff notice whether residents enjoy and eat their food, and do they take note of any comments?

71

- Is a member of staff allocated to help the more disabled and frail residents at mealtimes?
- Is the food cut up prior to being served for the blind, the partially paralysed, or residents with severe arthritis in their hands?
- Do you provide cutlery specifically designed for people with disabilities?
- Do staff hurry the residents through their meals in order to clear up quickly, or do they give them time to socialise with other residents and enjoy their food?

7.1   WEIGHT CHECKS

A resident will be weighed on their arrival at the care home. This will be recorded and then checked monthly. This is important because an unexplained weight gain or loss can indicate a health problem.

WEIGHT LOSS
This could indicate:

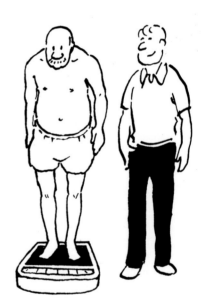

- illness or depression
- inadequate diet
- chewing and swallowing difficulties
- a problem with medication and/or drug therapy.

WEIGHT GAIN
This could indicate:

- overeating (or eating the incorrect type of food)
- insufficient exercise
- illness or depression
- a problem with medication and/drug therapy.

Residents most at risk are those who are admitted into the care home in a sick or frail condition, or who have been living alone. Their diet over the preceding months may have consisted of non-nutritious convenience

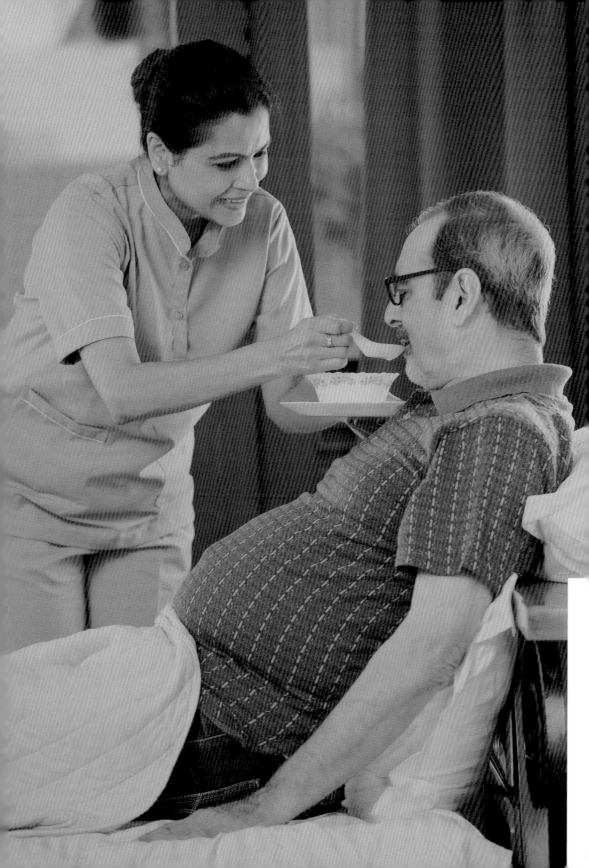

foods, or they may have had a problem with eating. This could be because of an issue with their mouth, such as badly fitting dentures or a sore tongue, difficulty with swallowing, or because they could not manage to shop or cook for themselves.

Care assistants must be very patient and understanding with these residents, particularly during the settling-in period. If their appetites is poor, it may be difficult to get them to eat properly at first. This can take quite a long time to achieve and must be done gradually.

Try not to press them to eat too much too quickly. Tempt them with their favourite dishes and always make sure that the food is high in nutrients. If a resident is forced to eat too much too quickly, it could give them indigestion and may put them off food altogether.

Patience and kindness during this period will bring very satisfying results to both the resident and the care assistant. Once the person is enjoying a full diet again, you should see them go from strength to strength.

8   FALLS AND BLACKOUTS

There are many reasons for falls and blackouts, and it is not the responsibility of the care assistant to diagnose them, but to report them to the manager when they occur.

Dizzy spells can be caused by a number of things, such as:

- inflammation in the ear
- a fall in blood pressure
- certain drugs
- alcohol
- the pulse becoming irregular, making the person feel faint.

Giddiness and unsteadiness can severely limit the amount of activity someone can do. It may be caused by a sudden movement such as getting up too quickly. Older people may find that it takes longer for them to adjust to a new position, such as bending down to tie up a shoelace, then standing up again. Residents should be encouraged to get up or out of bed more slowly, ideally in three stages:

- Sit up.
- Dangle the legs over the side of the bed.
- Stand up slowly.

A narrowing of the blood vessels in the neck, or arthritis in the neck, may also cause an elderly resident to become dizzy when moving their head up and down or from side to side. An acute onset of dizziness may cause the resident to fall, with the risk of breaking an arm or a leg or cracking a rib.

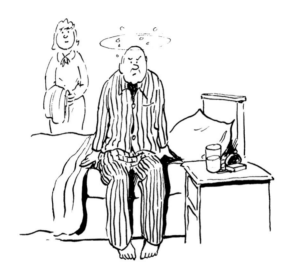

Remember, elderly people are often unable to get up after a fall without assistance and therefore it will be up to you to help them (see Section 5 on lifting). Before moving or lifting a resident, ensure that no bones are broken and that they have not damaged anything. If in doubt, inform your manager or senior carer on duty. It is wise to have the resident checked over by the GP, even if there does not seem to be any apparent injury.

It is a good idea for residents who are likely to fall to use a walking aid, such as a tripod or Zimmer. A soft collar for the neck may also help residents with arthritis or circulatory problems. These can be arranged through their GP, who should also be consulted if you and your manager are in any doubt as to what action to take.

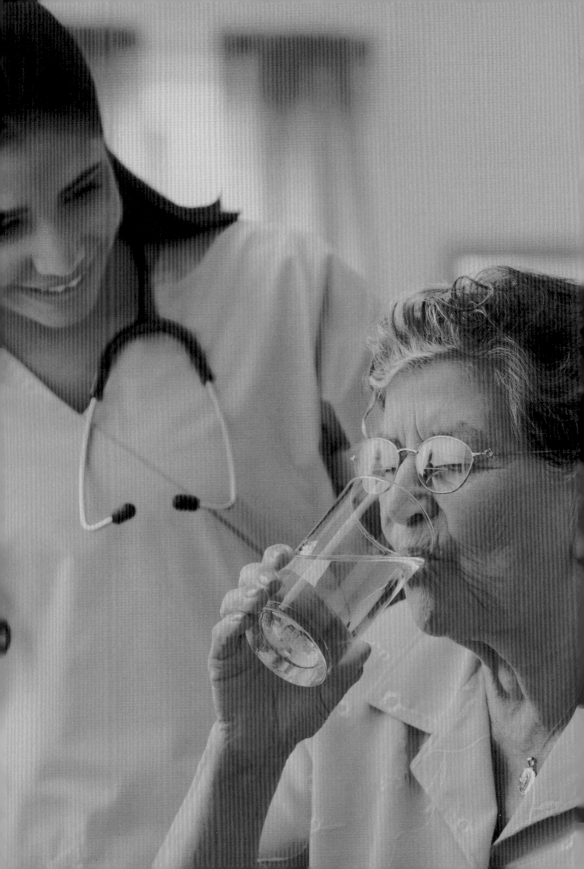

9   BLADDER AND BOWELS

9.1   CONSTIPATION

Constipation in the elderly may be caused by slower activity of the bowel, which results in incomplete emptying. Constipation is characterised by the passage of hard, dry faeces. It can also be caused by poor fluid intake and lack of exercise. The bowel may become blocked by a hard mass of faeces and the leakage of liquid material around this can occasionally give the appearance of diarrhoea. In this instance, contact the GP immediately.

Residents should be encouraged to drink at least three pints of liquid per day (preferably not of an alcoholic nature!). The correct diet, and eating enough dietary fibre, play an important part in preventing constipation.

If pure bran is used it should be taken with plenty of fluid. Too much bran can affect the absorption of some nutrients, e.g. zinc, calcium, iron.

Persistent difficulties of any kind with the bowel should be reported without delay to the GP. Prevention and treatment of constipation can be handled in a number of ways. Here are some useful tips:

- exercise
- high fibre diet
- plenty of fluids
- laxatives
- suppositories
- enemas.

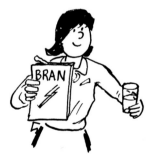
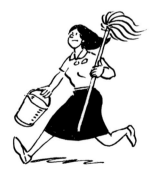

9.2 URINE INFECTIONS

Urine infections can be a common problem for the elderly and can have a dramatic effect on physical and mental wellbeing. It is important, therefore, to be aware of the early signs and symptoms. These generally show themselves in the following ways:

- Frequency: the resident will complain that they are passing urine very frequently.
- Pain: the resident will complain of pain when passing urine, but this is not always so.
- Colour/smell: the urine may be cloudy and have a distinctive smell.
- The resident may complain of general ill health and may be confused, or may suffer from incontinence.

Urine infections must be dealt with promptly. Inform the GP, who will leave a form and a bottle for you to collect a sample of urine (this is usually a mid-stream specimen and it must be collected in a sterile container). This is then sent for analysis. Once it has been analysed and the infection confirmed, the GP will prescribe the correct antibiotics.

Ideally, a further sample should be tested 14 days after the course of antibiotics has been completed, to confirm that the infection has cleared up. The likely treatments are:

- antibiotics
- plenty of fluids.

If a urine infection is left unchecked, then the acute condition could become chronic. This may result in:

- damaged kidneys
- incontinence
- confusion.

So take early action!

9.3 INCONTINENCE

It is impossible to understand the horror and shock that a person feels the first time they are incontinent. Their sense of humiliation and disgrace is difficult to appreciate without having experienced it yourself, therefore these residents need a special kind of understanding from the care assistant.

Your approach to them and your response to their plight can either destroy them or help them to understand what is happening. You can give the resident the encouragement and confidence to keep going.

Incontinence can be due to many causes, most of which, with the correct diagnosis and treatment, are curable. It can have a devastating effect on the life of the resident when it occurs, and can destroy their dignity and self-confidence. It is therefore vital that you take prompt action, so that the correct diagnosis can be made and treatment started as soon as possible. Do *not* let it go unchecked.

Incontinence is not merely a symptom of old age; there is always an underlying cause. You must have a positive approach to this condition and *not* accept the fact that it is simply part of growing old. It is not.

It is up to the care assistant to be aware of the possible causes and take immediate action if a resident suddenly starts to become incontinent. It's important for you to regularly ask them if they need assistance to get to the toilet.

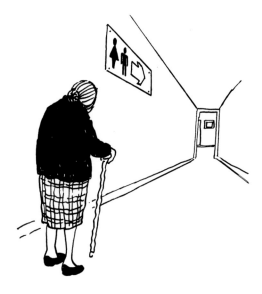

Possible causes of incontinence:

- Is the toilet too far away?
- Can the resident get out of their chair or bed easily to get to the toilet on time?
- Can they undo their clothes?
- Have they a urine infection?
- Are they constipated?
- Have they been prescribed any new drugs recently?
- If it's a man, has he got prostate trouble?
- Do they have a underlying physical disorder?
- Are they very depressed?
- Are they taking a too strong a sleeping tablet and not waking up in time?

The bladder is constantly being filled with urine from the kidneys and at the base of the bladder is a valve which is normally held shut. When the bladder fills, the pressure rises, the nerves send a message to the brain and you feel the need to pass water. In normal circumstances, a message is sent back from the brain at an appropriate time: the valve is then opened and the urine is passed out.

However, problems arise when the message is not passed or the valve itself becomes inefficient. This can be caused by an infection in the bladder, a mental disorder, depression or confusion, and sometimes drugs. Excitement can also have a similar effect.

Some residents have to take diuretic tablets. This increases the flow of urine from the kidneys to the bladder and therefore makes them have to pass water more frequently. Residents who are on these tablets are often afraid to drink, because they think that it will make their frequency worse. This is not the case, so you must encourage them to drink regularly to prevent dehydration. Often the disabled resident may find that they cannot get to the toilet on time, or perhaps when they do it is occupied. In these instances, if they don't have an en-suite bathroom, always offer to put a commode in their room.

If for any reason the incontinence cannot be resolved and is permanent, it is crucial that you have a proper routine for handling the condition. All staff must appreciate the devastating effect that incontinence can have on the resident, and handle it with understanding, discretion and professionalism. Your approach is vital in helping to restore the dignity and self-confidence of the resident.

Practical actions:

Make sure that the bed has a plastic mattress cover, plastic draw sheet and plastic pillow cover. This will reassure the resident that they are not damaging the bed. It is advisable to have drip-dry bed linen for easy maintenance. Bed linen should also be easy to wash and not need ironing.

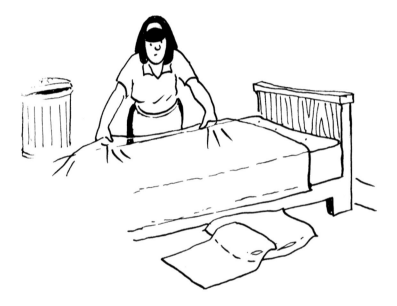

Keep a special large plastic dustbin in the laundry room, filled with water and disinfectant. Soiled linen and clothing can be placed in the dustbin for a 24 hours to be sterilised. Once a day, rinse through the contents, put them in the washing machine then refill the dustbin with a new solution of water and disinfectant. If this procedure is carried out regularly, it will ensure that no soiled linen or clothing is left lying about, which could cause cross-infection. Keep the home fresh by using air fresheners to combat any unwelcome smells.

Cleanliness is of paramount importance. Keep a supply of plastic bin liners handy in the laundry room for soiled incontinence pads. This way, the pads can be put straight into the liner and the bag removed. People's personal hygiene is very important, therefore daily baths or blanket baths are essential.

9.4   DEHYDRATION

Elderly people can very quickly become dehydrated and therefore need to be encouraged to drink plenty of fluids.

Below are some, but not all, of the possible causes of dehydration, together with the symptoms:

Causes:

- Certain medication, such as antibiotics or diuretics
- Alcohol
- Central heating and air conditioning
- Lack of fluid intake

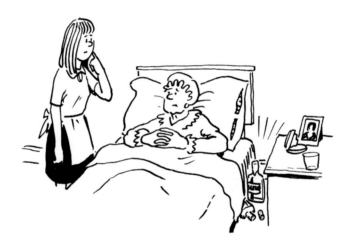

Signs and symptoms:

- Confusion
- Headaches
- Very dry and shrivelled skin with a loss of elasticity
- Constipation

If you spot these symptoms, the best course of action is to:

- Advise your manager, who will report it to the GP
- Increase the resident's fluid intake
- Start a fluid chart recording inputs and outputs
- Check what drugs the resident is on.

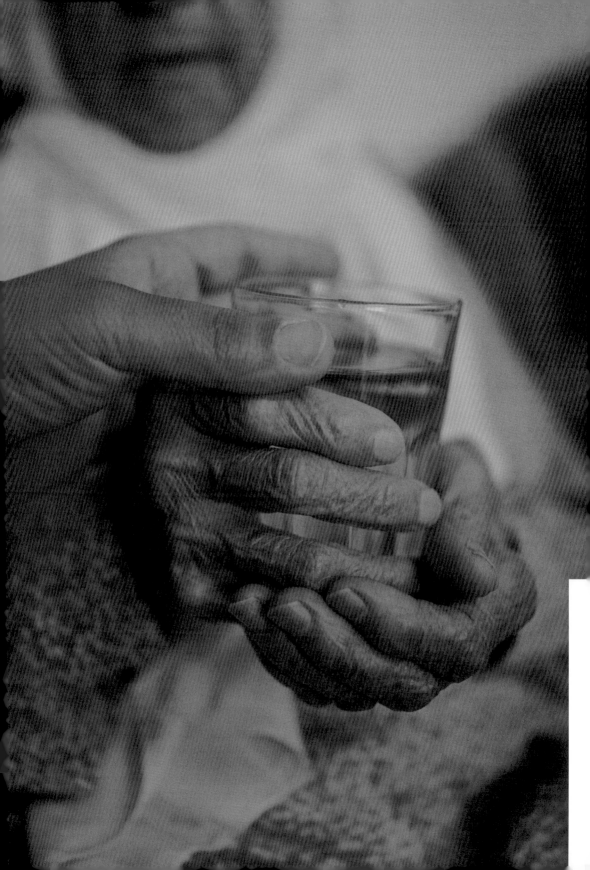

10 DEMENTIA AND CONFUSION

Dementia occurs when a person's brain starts to show signs of age. It can affect their memory, reasoning power and decision making. In most cases there is nothing to be alarmed about, but extra care may be needed. If you notice that a resident has any of the symptoms below, it is very important that you inform the manager, who will then contact the GP to arrange for tests to be carried out to get a diagnosis. Some of the symptoms are:

- depression
- forgetfulness
- constantly fretting
- confusion
- mood swings from one extreme to another
- wandering

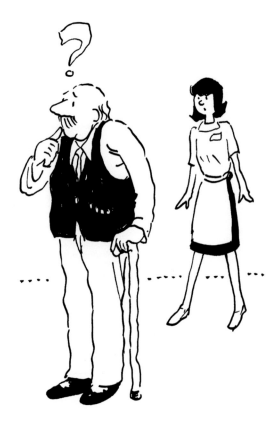

- anxiety and stress
- misplacing items
- poor appetite
- incontinence
- paranoid ideas and hallucinations.

A person with dementia may be confused for some, or all, of the time. Any sudden change in a resident's condition – either starting to be confused or getting more confused when normally they are in a mildly confused state – may be caused by the following:

- physical illness, such as an infection, particularly of the chest and bladder
- cardiac failure
- excessive or incorrect medication
- excessive night sedatives.

Should any of these symptoms become apparent, your manager must be informed, and the GP consulted.

11 WHAT TO DO IN AN EMERGENCY

HEALTH AND SAFETY—The best thing to do in an emergency is to be prepared. That is why you must read, understand and sign the Health and Safety manual. Your manager should explain your responsibilities to you in detail within a few weeks of you joining the home. This ensures that you are well informed and working in a safe and healthy environment. When accidents happen or an emergency arises, it is vital that you know what to do. The two types of emergency you may have to deal with are classified as medical and non-medical.

Medical emergencies are things like:

- falling
- bleeding
- choking.

Non-medical emergencies are things like:

- fire.

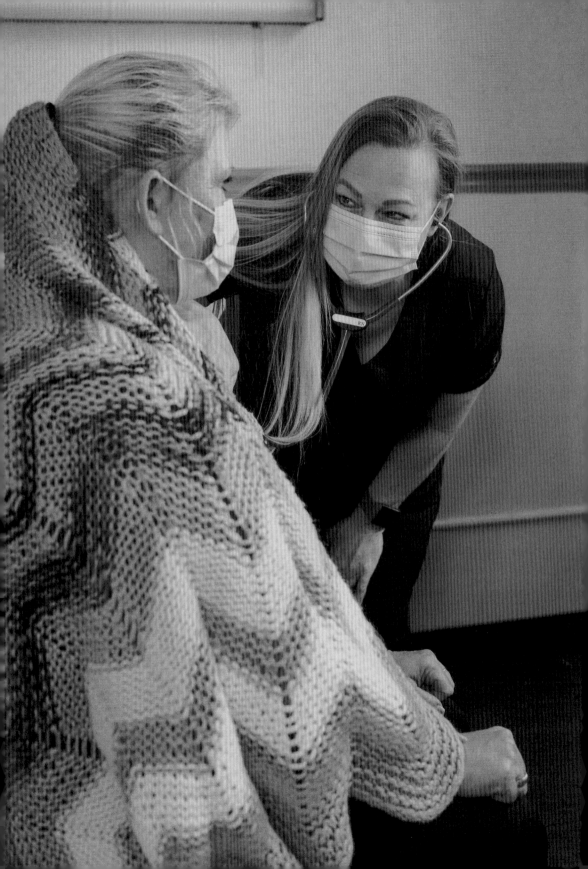

Fire, if you are not trained how to react when you find one, can lead to tragedy. Every year people die in fires in care homes. Dealing with a serious fire is one of the biggest challenges a care assistant will ever face, so it is very important that you are trained, so that you know what to do. Section 3 of this book deals with the prevention of fire as well as what to do in the event of a fire breaking out.

If you are faced with an emergency, remember the four As:

- Assessment
- Assistance
- Action
- Assurance.

12 INFECTION PREVENTION AND CONTROL

Since Covid-19 hit the UK at the beginning of 2020, care home staff have never had such an important role to play in the prevention and control of infections in their care home. It is therefore essential that their induction and ongoing training includes information on pandemics, infection, prevention and control as well as good personal hygiene practices.

Infectious diseases can spread readily to other residents and cause outbreaks within a care setting. The most common outbreaks are due to viral respiratory infections and gastroenteritis, and can be easily spread by hand-to-hand contact. Therefore, care staff should *not* wear rings (other than a plain smooth band), wristwatches or wrist jewellery.

Care staff should know how to wash their hands with soap and warm water, especially:

- before and after they have any contact with residents
- after contact with bodily fluid or secretions
- after handling soiled or contaminated equipment, clothes or bedding
- before eating, drinking or handling food
- after using the toilet
- after touching animals or animal foods.

12.1   PERSONAL PROTECTIVE EQUIPMENT (PPE)

Personal protective equipment (PPE) is used to protect staff while performing specific tasks. It includes gowns, gloves and masks, which are generally for single use. During an outbreak, staff must use appropriate PPE for their care procedures:

- non-sterile disposable gloves
- disposable plastic aprons
- hazardous waste bags – in a rigid container
- liquid soap and paper towels.

12.2   THE ENVIRONMENT

Keeping the environment clean is essential to reducing the spread of infection in care homes. Your manager will brief the cleaning staff about the infection outbreak and ensure they are trained and supported to carry out their duties, including how to protect themselves.

During an infection outbreak, the manager will increase the frequency of cleaning until the last affected person is symptom-free. Cleaning and decontamination must be performed by staff who have been trained in the use of appropriate PPE and disinfectant. Below are the cleaning tasks and schedules that *must* be carried out:

- Hard surfaces should be disinfected at least once a day.
- Handrails, door handles, toilet rails, bath rails and taps must be cleaned with disinfectant at least three times a day.
- Equipment such as commodes should be thoroughly cleaned with detergent and hot water after each use.
- Windows should be kept open for as long as possible, to allow ventilation of an infected area.
- Soft furnishings should be thoroughly steam-cleaned in the affected unit or areas.

12.3   LINEN AND LAUNDRY

Care homes use a variety of laundry systems and equipment, so it is important for you to understand the system being used in yours. Correct handling and storage of linen, including bed sheets, towels and clothing, is essential as they can carry infection. Always wear gloves and an apron when you handle laundry. Here are some tips:

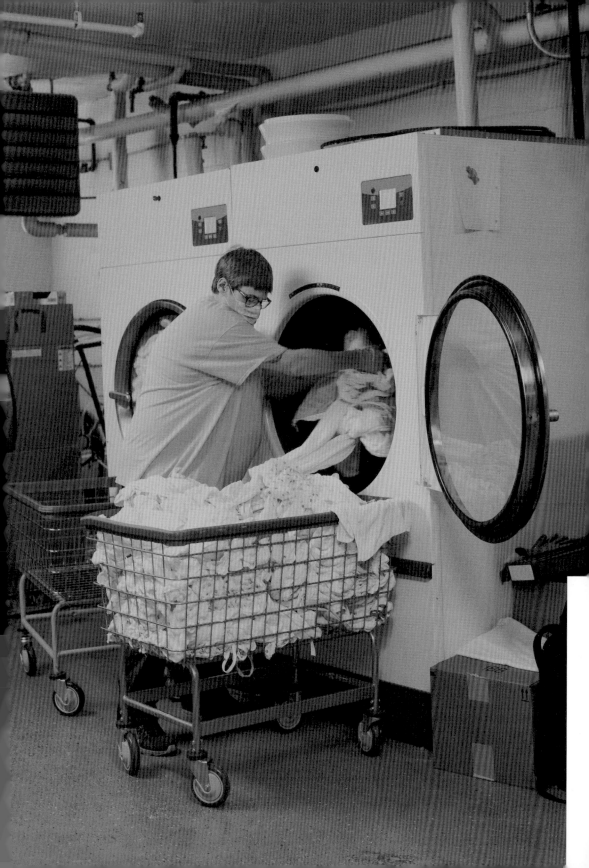

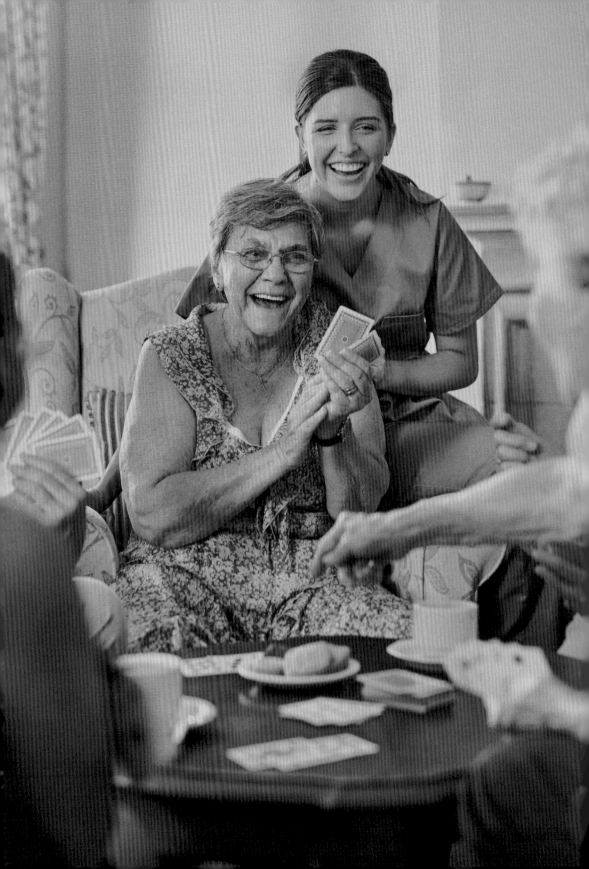

- Treat all linen as infected if a resident is known to have an infectious illness.
- Do not perform manual sluicing of laundry.
- Segregate laundry appropriately.
- Wash all linen and clothing in a dedicated laundry room, using the correct procedures.
- Keep all laundry in bags or baskets, not loose on the floor.
- Store laundry in a dry area above floor level, not with used linen.
- Use different trolleys for clean, used and soiled laundry, to avoid cross-contamination.

13 SO, YOU THINK YOU CAN DO THE JOB?

At the start of this book, we said that your job as a care assistant was to help your residents to take better care of themselves. But as we've seen, that's not always as easy as it sounds. Your job as a carer is a very demanding one, which requires many skills in a lot of different areas which always have to be delivered with patience and understanding. However, you will find it difficult to find a more rewarding and fulfilling career.

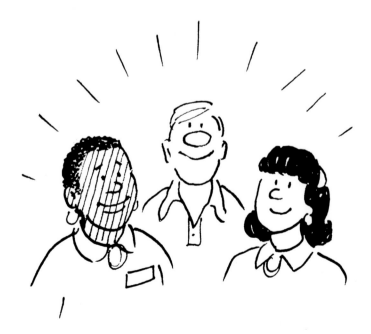

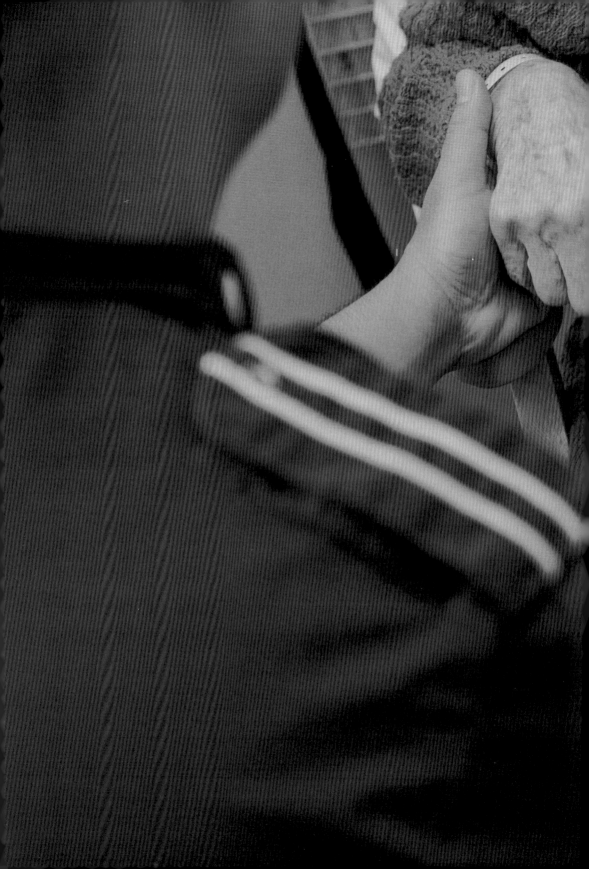

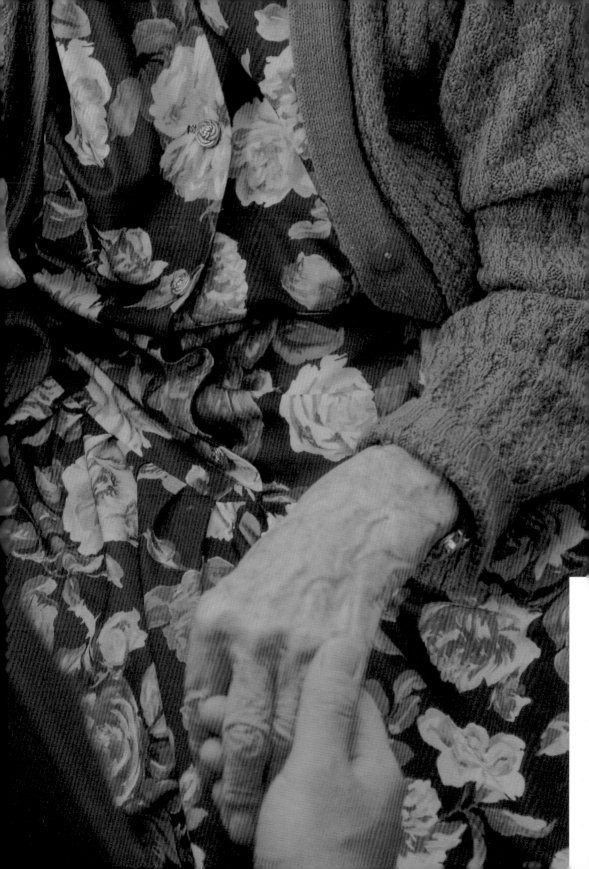

NOTES

M	T	W

PLANNER

T	F	S / S

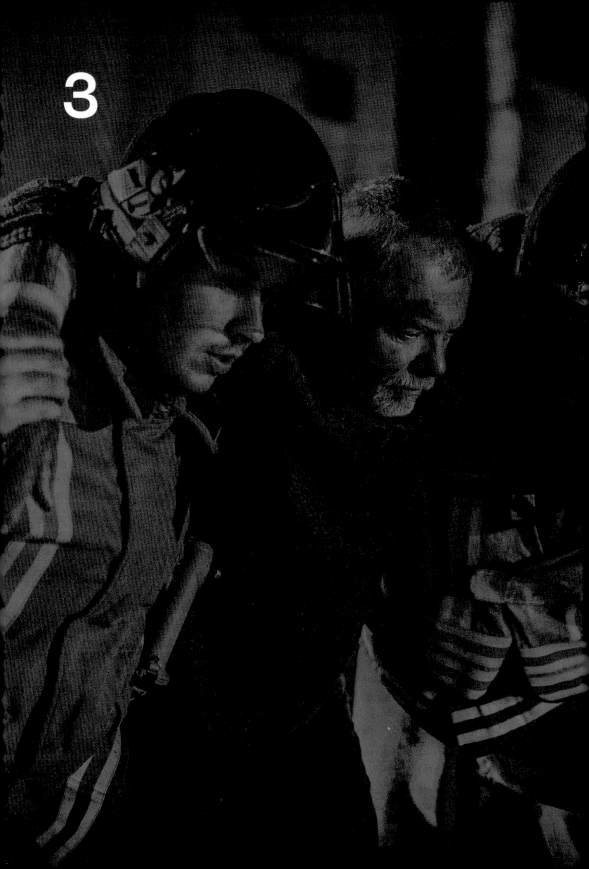

FIRE TRAINING

1 INTRODUCTION

All residential care homes must comply with the Statutory Fire Safety Regulations before they can be registered by the regulator.

The introduction of the Regulatory Reform (Fire Safety) Order 2005 (The Fire Safety Order) was the biggest change in fire safety legislation for more than 30 years. This collates the fire safety requirements from approximately 118 pieces of legislation and brings them together under one umbrella.

You may be sitting reading this book in a room in the building in which you work, wondering how this may apply to you. If so, you should know that under this new legislation you have some responsibility for the safety of the people in the premises, including residents and colleagues. You also have a responsibility to assist the 'responsible person' by ensuring that the fire preventive and protective measures provided in the building are functioning effectively.

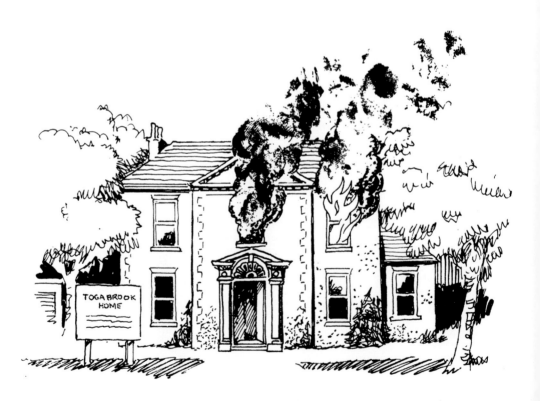

Every year people die in fires in care homes. Dealing with a serious fire is one of the biggest challenges a care assistant will ever face. If you act incorrectly during a fire, it may cost your life or someone else's. All fires are different and so the basic rules in this booklet must become second nature to you. This will enable you to fulfil your responsibilities effectively, providing you know exactly how to respond when the fire alarm bell rings.

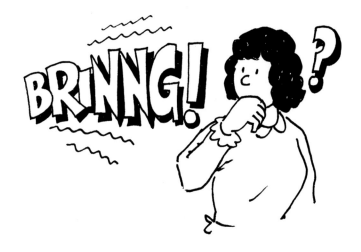

This section of the book is divided into the following five parts. They will help you to understand your practical responsibilities relating to any fire emergency:

HOW FIRES START AND SPREAD

HOW YOUR BUILDING IS PROTECTED AGAINST FIRE

RAISING THE ALARM

EVACUATING THE BUILDING

STAYING PREPARED

When dealing with a fire, the most important thing to remember is:
DON'T PANIC.

2   HOW FIRES START AND SPREAD

The most common causes of fire are:

- cooking, especially deep fat frying
- smoking
- deliberate ignition (arson)
- electric heaters
- electrical faults.

  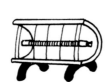 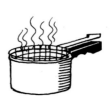 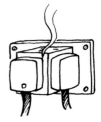

Here are a few tips and hints:

- Disconnect (or switch off at the socket) all electrical apparatus when not in use.
- Check that small portable appliances are not showing any signs of wear and tear, e.g. frayed or damaged cables, cracked plugs or decolourisation due to overheating.
- Do not leave combustible rubbish or flammable substances like spray cans of furniture polish and other cleaning fluids lying around.
- Disconnect electric underblankets before beds are occupied.
- Empty wastepaper baskets regularly.
- Make sure that electric radiant bar heaters cannot be placed too close to items that may catch fire, e.g. upholstered furniture or curtains.
- If you suspect a that resident is smoking in bed, look for signs and report them to your manager (this is particularly important for staff who work at night).

How to deal with a chip pan fire:

- Call the fire brigade.
- Don't move the pan.
- Turn off the heat, if you can do this safely.

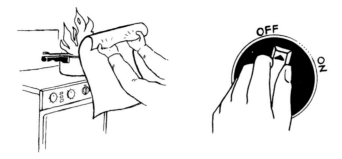

- Protecting your hands, place a fire blanket, damp cloth or close-fitting lid over the pan to smother the flames.
- Leave the pan to cool for at least 30 minutes. The fire can start again if the cover is removed too soon.
- NEVER PUT WATER ON THE FIRE.

Fire needs three components to exist. This is often referred to as the *triangle of fire.*

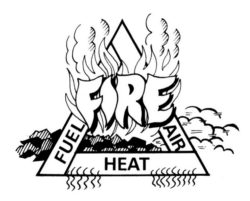

Remove any one of these components and the fire will go out. As a fire grows it produces heat, flames and smoke.

2.1   HOW FIRES SPREAD

SMOKE is the biggest killer in fires. It spreads around the building, making it difficult to see, and quickly asphyxiates its victims. Because smoke is hot, it rises and tends to fill a room or corridor from the ceiling down. A fire in a single room can generate enormous volumes of smoke and toxic gases, which can reach temperatures of more than 1,000°C, and can kill anyone who breathes in the smoke.

But smoke has an enemy: the door.

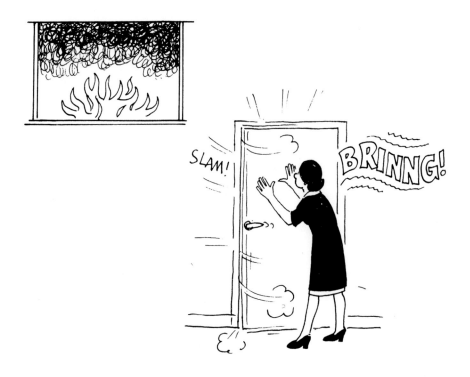

FIRE DOORS are essential as they are fitted with smoke seals, which contain the smoke and hot gases in the room where the fire originated, leaving corridors and stairwells clear so that people can escape safely. Fire doors must be kept closed at all times, especially at night, so that deadly smoke cannot travel from one room to another.

If a fire door has to be kept open for a specific reason, an approved fire door hold-open device must be fitted: these allows doors to close automatically when the fire alarm goes off. If you see fire doors wedged open or furniture in corridors as you move around the home, immediately report it to your manager.

Here are a few tips and hints:

- If there is a fire in the vicinity, do not open windows as this will let in oxygen, which will feed the fire.
- Be very careful about opening the door to a room that may be on fire.
- Listen for the sound of burning, or for ornaments and other objects falling. Touch the door handle briefly with the back of your hand to

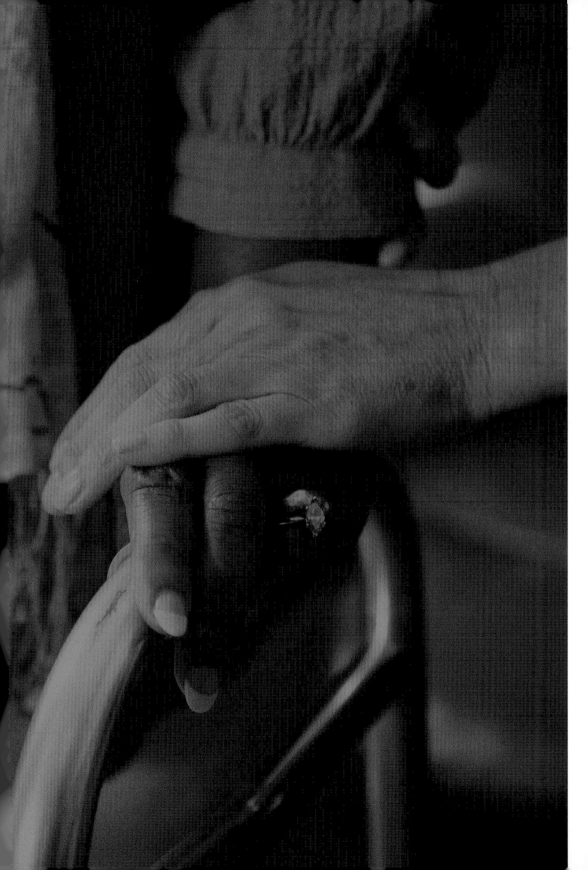

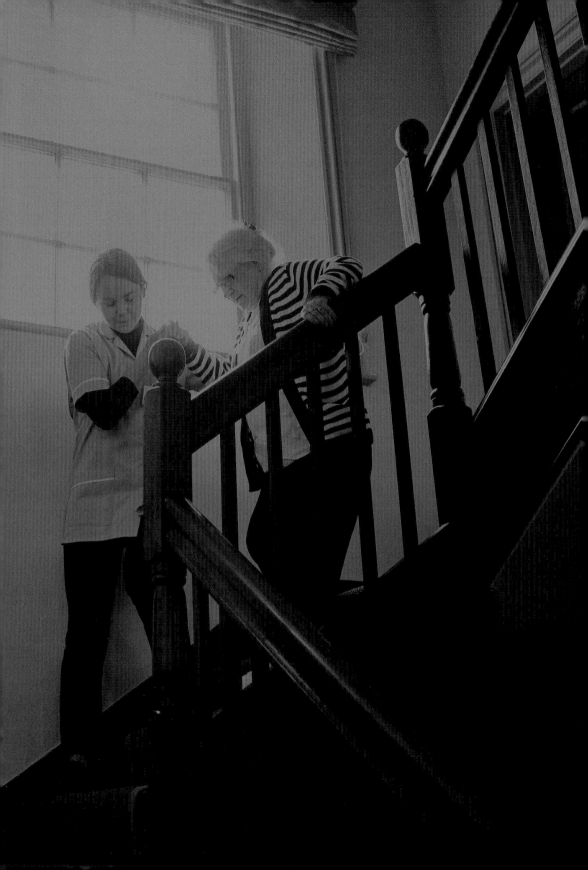

test whether it is hot. If you even suspect that there may be a fire in the room, leave the door closed and raise the alarm.
- If you do encounter smoke, keep low. The cleanest, coolest air is always to be found at floor level and this will help to keep you alive.
- Direct others to get down into the clean air at floor level as well.
- Do not let anyone use the lift.

3 HOW YOUR BUILDING IS PROTECTED AGAINST FIRE

Management are responsible for organising a competent person to carry out an annual fire risk assessment, which includes inspecting the property and training the staff. A report is produced which must be actioned. The 'responsible person' is also required to carry out all fire drills and equipment tests and log them in the fire safety logbook:

- Annual tests of the fire alarm system are carried out and recorded.
- Weekly fire alarm tests.
- Three-monthly tests of the emergency lighting system.
- Three-monthly fire drills are carried out and recorded.
- Annual tests of the fire extinguishers.
- Safe exit routes are identified.
- Clear fire exit and directional signs are in place.
- Regular tests of all fire equipment. These should be done by suitably competent companies or individuals.

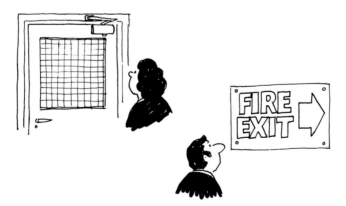

A few tips and hints:

- Make sure all fire doors are kept closed, especially at night.
- Make sure all corridors are kept clear of furniture and other combustible materials.
- Check that the emergency exit doors leading to the outside can open without needing a key and are unobstructed.

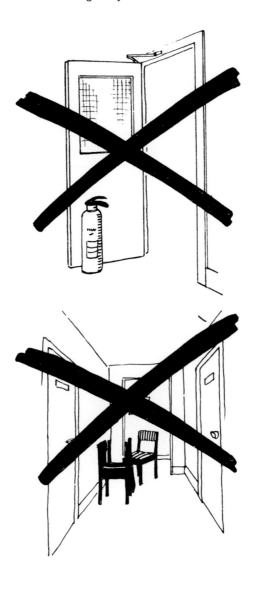

What about all the fire safety equipment we have mentioned? What does it all do? Let's follow the early stages of a fire to see the function each item fulfils.

- A fire starts in a bedroom.
- A smoke detector senses it and operates the fire alarm system.
- The location of the fire appears in the form of an illuminated light on the fire alarm panel.
- A power failure cuts off the electrical supply to the building, causing failure of the primary (normal) lighting and power circuits.
- Battery-powered emergency lighting units come on and illuminate the escape corridors, staircases, reception rooms and hallways.
- The fire alarm system, which also has a back-up battery supply, continues to sound.

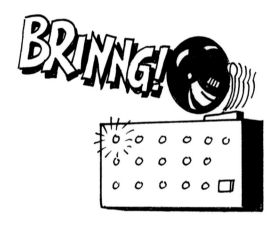

And of course, there are fire extinguishers.

Fire extinguishers are there to save the building, not the people, so remember to put people first. If one extinguisher doesn't put out the fire, get everyone out as quickly as possible, starting with those most at risk.

There are lots of different sorts of fire extinguishers, but the ones you are most likely to find in your care home are:

- water extinguishers
- dry powder extinguishers
- carbon dioxide (CO_2) extinguishers
- fire blankets.

Generally speaking, the best extinguisher is the nearest extinguisher, but there are a few exceptions.

Here's a guide to enable you to choose the most effective extinguisher for your situation. There are five colours/types of extinguisher:

- RED (Water) – to be used on fires involving wood, paper, textiles, furniture, beds, bedding

- BLUE (Dry powder) – to be used on fires involving electrical items or flammable liquids

- CREAM (Foam) – to be used on fires involving flammable liquids like petrol and paraffin

- BLACK (Carbon dioxide, CO_2) – to be used on fires involving electrical items or flammable liquids

- YELLOW (Wet chemical)– to be used on fires involving chip pan and deep fat fryers

- FIRE BLANKET – To be used on chip pan fires or when clothing is on fire

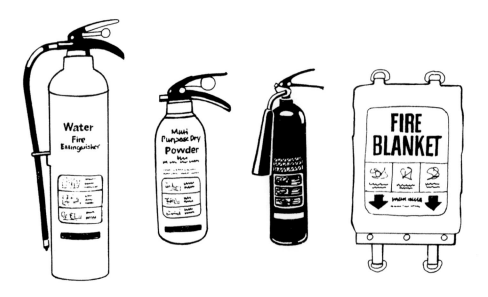

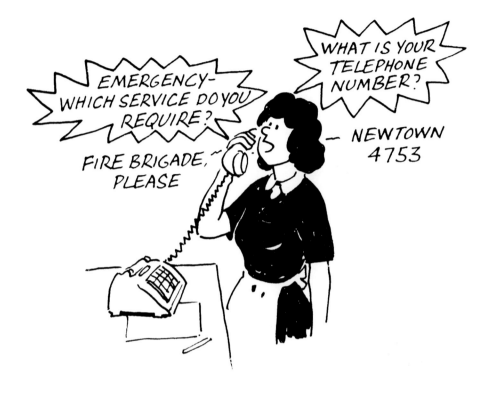

4   RAISING THE ALARM

This either happens automatically, when smoke or heat from the fire activates a detector head, which sets off the alarm, or it can be carried out manually by operating one of the fire alarm call points.

Next, you or a colleague must dial 999. Do not think twice about dialling 999 and never assume that a colleague has already done it. The fire brigade don't mind being called out, even for the smallest of fires. It is part of your responsibility to make sure they are on their way.

Things that you need to do straightaway are:

- Check the location of the fire on the alarm panel.
- Make sure someone has called the fire brigade.
- Unlock the front door but keep it closed, so that the fire crews can have access when they arrive.

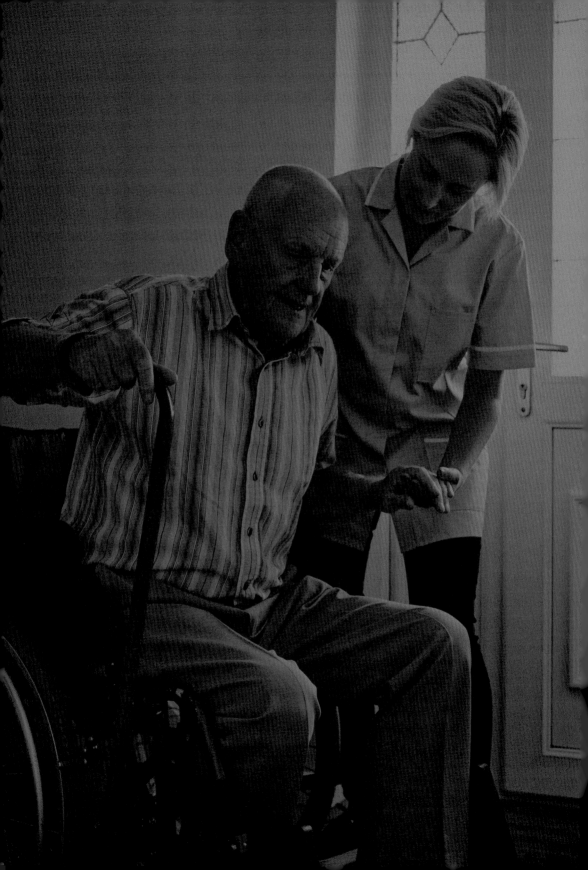

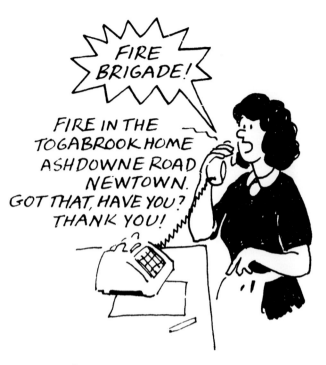

So, to recap, you must:

- Raise the alarm.
- Ring the fire brigade.
- Get immediate help.

Tips and hints:

- The only phone call that you must make immediately is to the emergency services. Do not call the proprietor.
- Even if you do nothing else, always dial 999.

When you make a 999 call, the operator will need to know certain things clearly and quickly. They will want to know:

- Your phone number.
- Whether you need the fire and rescue service, police or ambulance service.
- How many people there are in the building.

This information will be used to assess how many and what types of fire engines should attend. It may also be used to indicate whether the ambulance service and/or police should also attend.

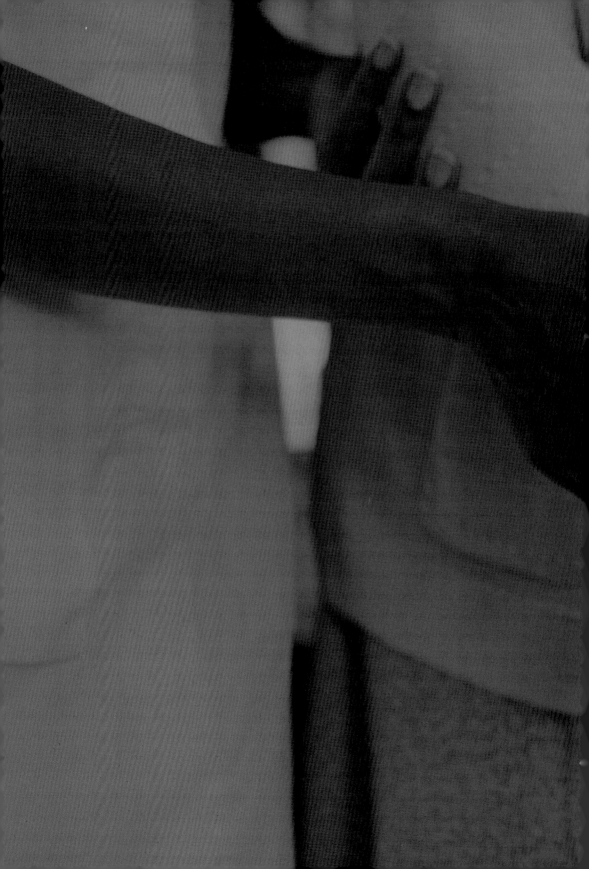

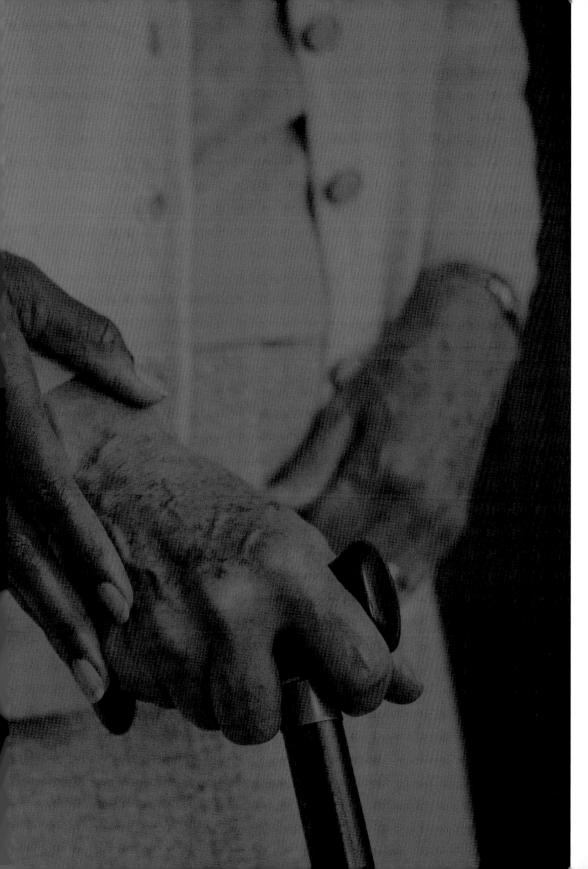

5 EVACUATING THE BUILDING

- Ensure each resident's Personal Emergency Evacuation Procedure (PEEP) form is available.

- Go to the area where the fire is.

- Start evacuating people nearest to the fire.

- Evacuate them to the designated area in the evacuation plan.

A few tips and hints:

- Get on with the evacuation as quickly as possible.
- Always investigate the area of a suspected fire in pairs; never go alone.
- Approach any door that opens into an area where you believe there may be a fire with extreme caution. If you feel heat, smell smoke or hear the sound of burning, don't open it.
- Close doors and windows wherever possible.
- Get the more alert residents to help the less mobile or motivated ones.
- Motivate people to move. Elderly people may not understand the urgency in fire situations.
- Leave people who are the most difficult to move until last unless they are in the immediate vicinity of the fire.

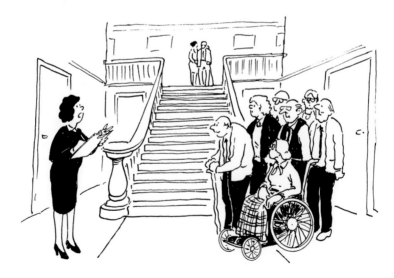

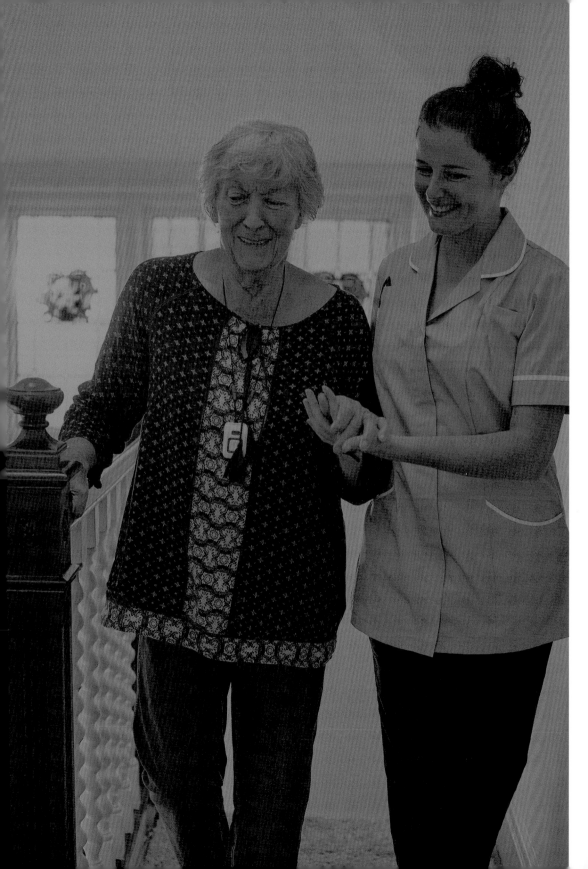

5.1   DANGERS

- Don't panic, otherwise you may make the wrong decision.
- Hot toxic smoke will be spreading throughout the building so remember to close all the doors.
- Flashovers. Sometimes heat can build up in a room and produce unburned gases. Don't open the door or a wall of flame could engulf you. If you do touch a door to see whether it is hot because there might be a fire behind it, touch it with the back of your hand. That way, if your hand gets burned you will still be able to use it afterwards.
- Hot door handles: again, feel these with the back of your hand.

5.2   MOVING IMMOBILE RESIDENTS

The various methods of moving immobile residents should only be attempted if you have been properly trained in the necessary techniques, to ensure you do not injure yourself or those you are helping.

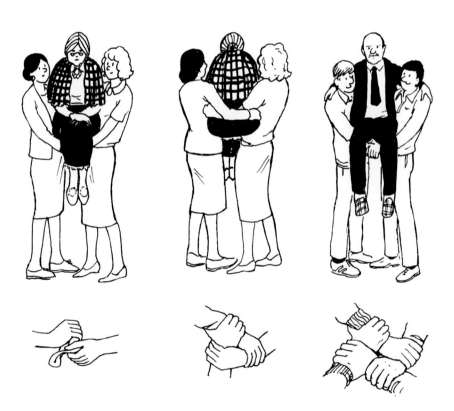

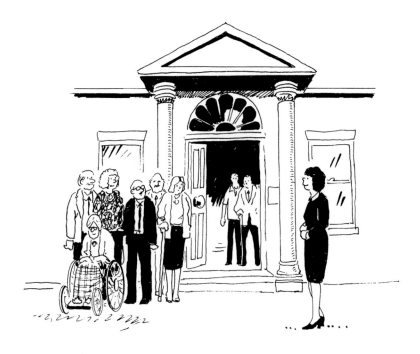

A few tips and hints:

- Some people get violent when they panic; don't let them injure you. You are only useful to the other residents if you are fully functional.
- When you are making your mental roll call of where everybody is, double-check against a printed list. (A printed list of all residents and staff should be available as part of the evacuation procedure).
- GET PEOPLE TO A PLACE OF SAFETY, STARTING WITH THOSE CLOSEST TO THE FIRE, AS THEY ARE MOST AT RISK.

The fire brigade will let you know of their arrival by sounding their sirens as they approach. Make sure someone meets them at or near the front door to brief them on the fire situation and to give them whatever further information they ask for:

- Where the fire is.
- How many people are still inside the building and where they are likely to be found.
- Residents' completed PEEP forms.

Now your job is over. NEVER GO BACK INTO A FIRE.

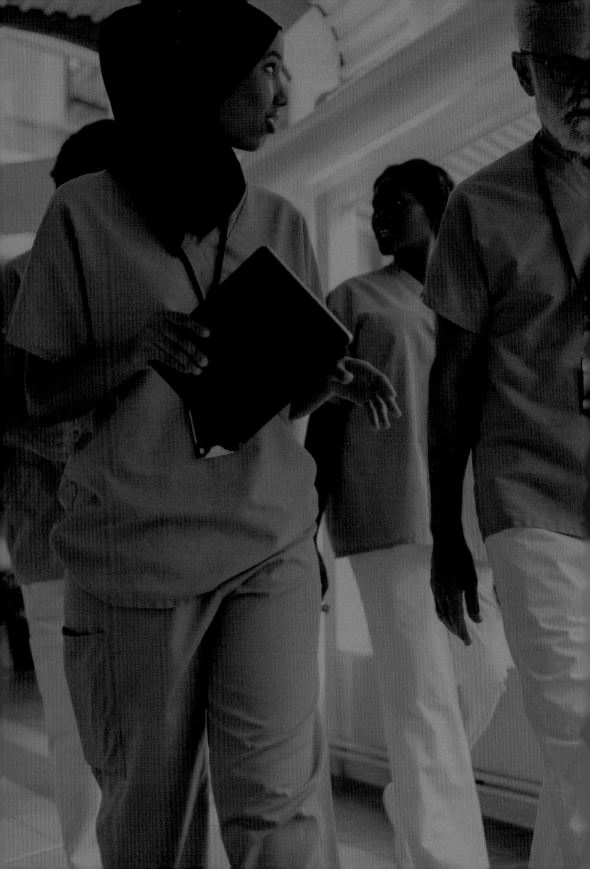

6 STAYING PREPARED

If you make a mistake during a fire it may cost your life or someone else's. All fires are different. The basic rules in the book must become second nature to you if you are able to fulfil your responsibilities under the Fire Safety Order. So, what should you do?

Practice makes perfect, and that means:

- Regular fire drills, at least twice a year.
- Regular tests of all fire equipment. These should be done by competent contractors. On-site staff should test the alarms weekly and the emergency lighting every month.
- All drills and equipment tests should be logged in a fire safety logbook.

The fire drills should simulate conditions in which one or more of the escape routes are obstructed by smoke. Put up signs stating 'Not this way' so that all residents have to use an alternative escape route.

As far as practicable, all people in the building should take part in the fire drills. Where people have not been able to take part in a drill for some reason, they should be taken around the building on another occasion to re-familiarise them with the escape routes.

Remember that all fires and fire drills are a race against time.

And good luck. You'll need it, even if you are fully prepared.

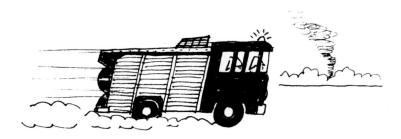

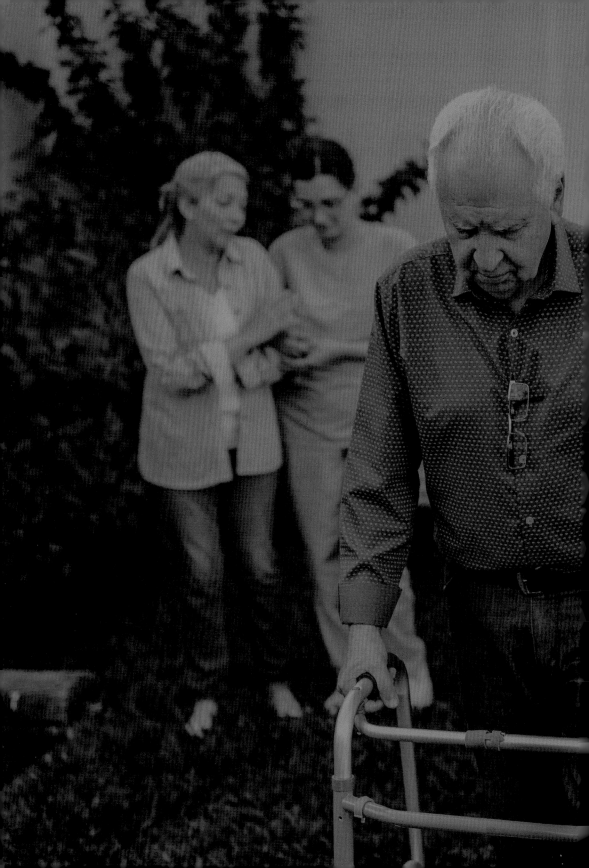

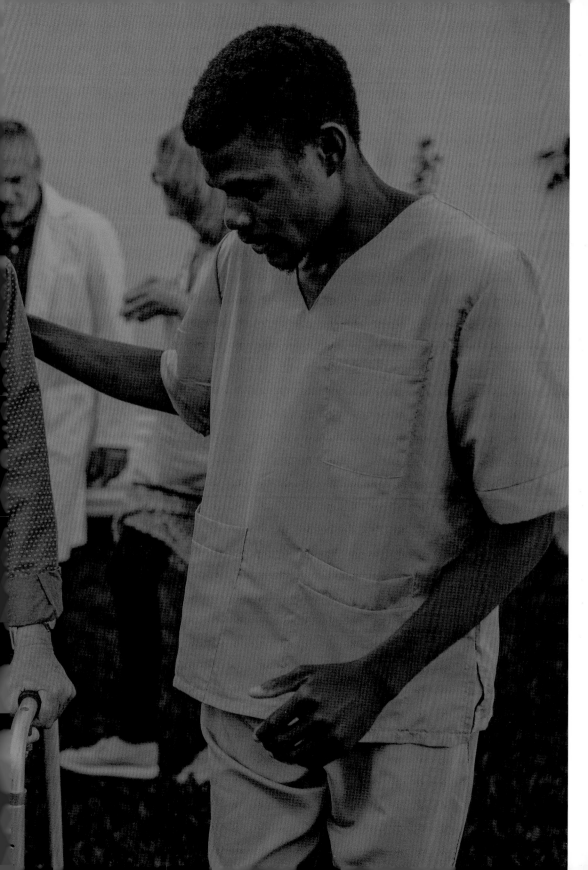

NOTES

FIRE TRAINING

NOTES

NOTES

FIRE TRAINING

M	T	W

T	F	S / S

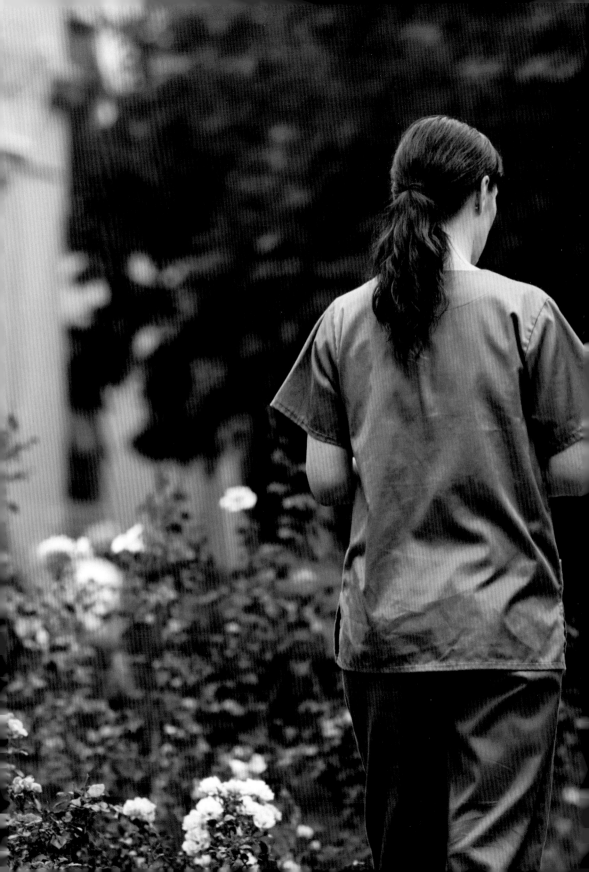

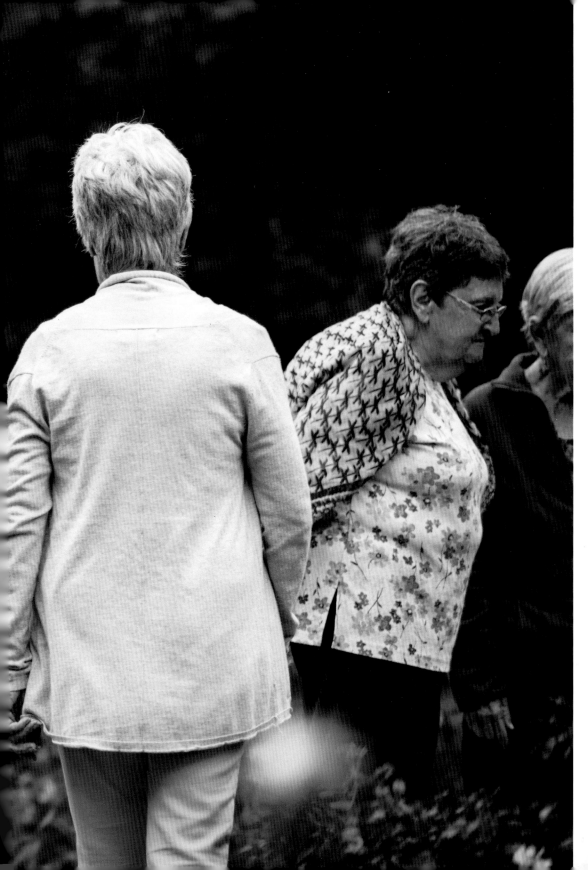

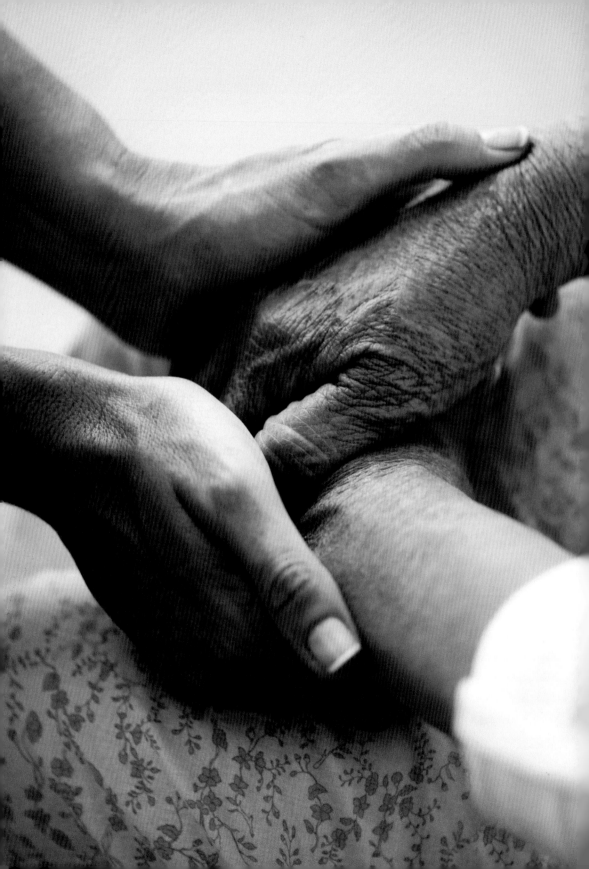

BIOGRAPHICAL NOTE

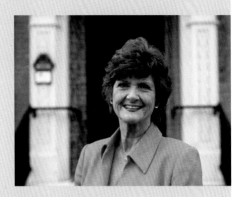

ABOUT THE AUTHOR

Sue Brand is Managing Director of RDB Star Rating. She trained and qualified at the Middlesex Hospital in London and started the Pembroke Group, her own group of care homes, in the 1970s. She has always been committed to quality care, pioneering the first training videos and books designed for the care sector in 1987. She was Chair of East Sussex National Care Association and Brighton and Hove National Care Homes Association from 1992 to 2000, when the care sector was in crisis. To address the serious issues facing the care sector at that time, she founded the RDB Star Rating System.

Sue has always been passionate about residents being treated with dignity and respect, and has spent many years campaigning to achieve this. She is very focused and highly tenacious, using her significant experience, intellectual abilities, and interpersonal skills to ensure that her objectives for quality care are reached and surpassed.

Current activities:

- Fellow of the Royal Society of Arts
- Founder member of the National Skills Academy
- Represents Care England on the UKAS Policy Advisory Council
- Member of the drafting panel of the British Standards Institute (BSI) for Social Care
- Member of the Royal Society of Medicine
- Trustee of the National Dignity Council
- Board member of the Quality Care Campaign
- Member of the Health and Social Care Accreditation Forum (HASCAF)
- Cranfield alumnus
- Common Purpose alumnus

ABOUT RDB STAR RATING

RDB Star Rating is an independent quality inspection company, committed to driving up standards in social care by carrying out annual inspections to enhance transparency to prospective customers.

The RDB model and assessment tool is client focused, holistic, objective and developmental in its approach. It encompasses a diverse range of care standards, varying from the way personal care is delivered to the management of the home and its personnel.

Care homes are evaluated against more than 200 RDB care standards, which are drawn from best practice research across the care sector and tempered by what is realistic and achievable, reflecting what good providers do naturally. Ten to 16 items of evidence are collected for each standard, from residents, management, staff and documentation, and 25 of the key standards are underpinned with a quality assurance standard.

Homes receive a report which includes graphs depicting their overall performance, their performance for each standard, and the results of their confidential resident and staff satisfaction surveys.

RDB products and assessments are based on the principles of best practice benchmarking and are certified by the United Kingdom Accreditation Service (UKAS), to the international and European standard ISO/IEC 17020:2012 for inspection bodies. RDB was the first company in the UK to achieve this award for social care.

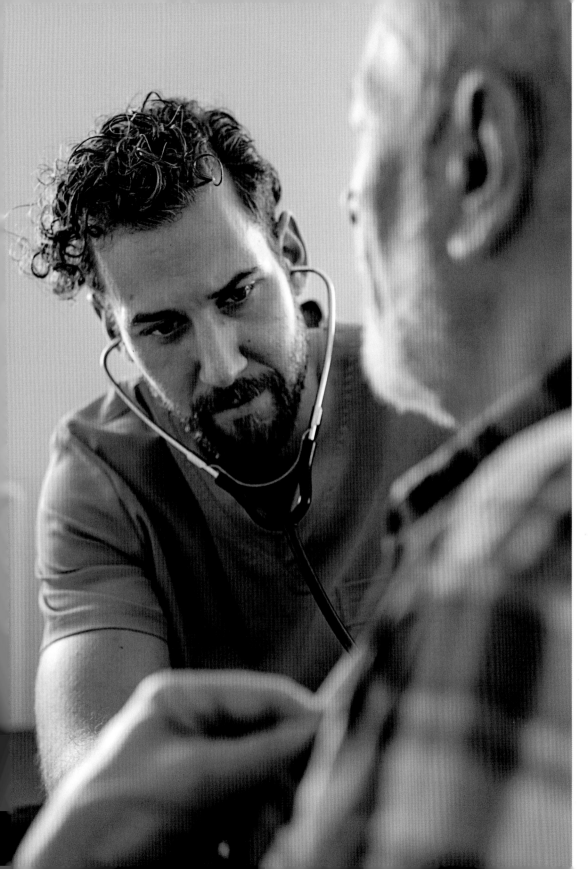

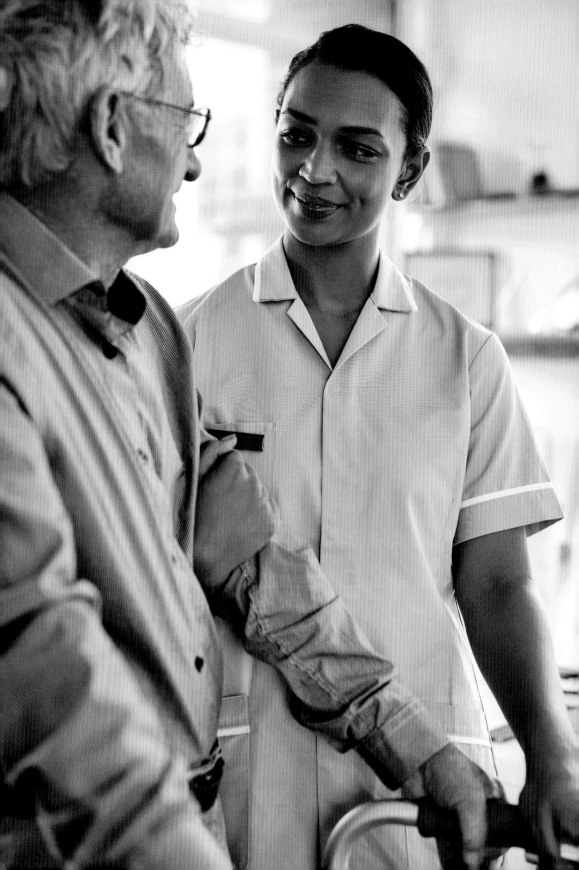

ACKNOWLEDGEMENTS

In memory of my brother-in-law Dr Peter Walden MRCP, who died on 15 January 2021.

I would like to thank my wonderful husband, who has supported me throughout our journey from the very first time we met while I was training to be a nurse at the Middlesex Hospital. I would also like to thank our two children, Nicholas and Joanna, and our delightful granddaughter Matty for their continued love and support.

It has been a great privilege for me to work in the care sector all my working life and to meet so many amazing and dedicated people with the same goal: to improve the quality of life for those who need it most.

There are too many individuals to acknowledge. I'm truly indebted to those of you who are mentioned, and can never thank you enough for your kindness and willingness to help and support me.

Firstly, I should like to give a special thanks to Manzoor Ishani, our great friend and solicitor who has guided me throughout the years. Deepest gratitude to the UKAS team for their support: Lord Lindsay Chairman, Matt Gantley CEO, Lorraine Turner, Stephen Mitchell, Louise Sanders and Professor Deborah Sturdy OBE; Professor Martin Green OBE and his dedicated team at Care England; Lord Blunkett, Lord Pickles, the Parliamentary Trust and Parliamentary Revue; Paul Stennett, Frank Alison, David Waters, Alison Wood, Jeremy Allin, and Peter Gross; Allan Bowman and the Brighton & Hove City Council.

A note of appreciation to the publisher, St James's House, particularly to Anna Danby, Publishing Director; Daphne Fordham-Smith, who provided efficient and friendly project management, Rachel Pfleger for her graphic design; and a special thanks to Darren Winter.

This book is published by St James's House, registered as a company in England and Wales as Regal Press Limited with company number 04132980. St James's House is an imprint within the SJH Group. Copyright is owned by the SJH Group.

St James's House   +44 (0)20 8371 4000
298 Regents Park Road   publishing@stjamess.org
London N3 2SZ   www.stjamess.org
United Kingdom

ISBN 978-1-906670-92-4

All information in this publication is verified to the best of the author's and publisher's ability. However, St James's House and the SJH Group do not accept responsibility for any loss arising from reliance on it. Where opinion is expressed, it is that of the author and does not necessarily coincide with the editorial views of the publisher.

The publishers have made all reasonable efforts to trace the copyright owners of the images reproduced herein, and to provide an appropriate acknowledgement in the book.

Cover photography by sturti/e+ via Getty Images.

Interior photography by Comstock/Stockbyte, Jacobs Stock Photography Ltd/Jose Luis Pelaez Inc/DigitalVision, Goodboy Picture Company/fstop123/PeopleImages/shapecharge/Dean Mitchell/sturti/PixelsEffect/Adene Sanchez/triloks/mixetto/RichLegg/wanderluster/simonkr/E+, Richard Bailey/Corbis Documentary, Jasmin Merdan/Jordan, Maskot/Maskot via Getty Images and DCPhoto/Dmytro Zinkevych via Alamy.

Printed in the UK by DG3 Leycol.

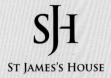

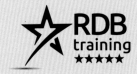